THE

WORKING

TRIATHLETE

MAXIMUM PERFORMANCE WITH BRUTAL EFFICIENCY

By Conrad Goeringer

Acknowledgements

This book would not have been possible without the editorial prowess of Alex and all the coaches, mentors and athletes I've had the privilege of working with over the last two decades.

Preface

Who are you?

If you are reading this book, you are likely a working professional with a rich life who either has a budding or mature interest in triathlon. You have a plethora of responsibilities apart from training, including family, work and travel. Add the prospect of high-level triathlon training on top of all that and you might be wondering if you will ever get the chance to sleep again. And — what's amusing — if you are like many triathletes, you may be rationalizing the prospect of not sleeping again. We are a hardcore bunch.

If you have spent time around triathletes, you probably have noticed the high occurrence of type-A personality types within the community. Yes, there are laid-back triathletes who do not care about performance, but relative to participants in other sports, triathletes are fiercely goal-oriented. Assuming you fit the mold, you are likely the kind of person who, when you set out to do something, does it (and not just for completion, but for dominance). You don't know how to function in any other way and that is generally a good thing; however, when you have numerous goals, pursuits and relationships to chase and cultivate simultaneously, your ability to grow in each of those areas is stifled. This is often an issue for triathletes, especially those who feel as if they need to train an inordinate number of hours per week to be competitive. "Sorry Johnny, I can't drive you to baseball practice this morning because I have to ride my bike for seven hours" is not something you should have to say to your kid. When you try to tackle too many things and do them well, you end up not doing any of them well, and your family, friends, employees or co-workers will grow to resent you.

There are two solutions to this common problem of wanting to do too much in too little time: (1) Eliminate or alter your goals (you probably do not want to do this) (2) Pursue your goals more efficiently (you probably want to do this).

If you are like most high-achieving individuals, you do not want to compromise performance goals. You want to push your limits and complete races as fast as your potential allows. Nonetheless, you realize that there is more to life than just triathlon and that committing an excessive amount of time to the sport can jeopardize your other ambitions. If you want to excel in all areas of your life, then you need an efficient roadmap to help you achieve more in fewer hours and – insofar as triathlon training goes — this book will help you do just that.

Why I wrote this book

As a passionate coach, triathlete and professional, I've always been interested in people who achieve in athletics, business, or otherwise. One common trait that successful people have is their ability to accomplish more in less time. Yes, you can get there with brute force, but the best way to excel in any given field is via focused practice and execution. The same concept can be applied to triathlon.

I wrote Working Triathlete to convey principles and strategies that allow the motivated working athlete to achieve more in less time. The focus is not on creating a gentle or easy training plan — it is on creating an efficient one that, by distilling the most essential training principles and time management hacks, will equip you with the tools to become a better (i.e., faster) triathlete.

As a coach, I get tremendous joy helping others break through their perceived limitations. I know what it is like to juggle numerous responsibilities while still putting in the work to perform at a high level and I consider it an honor to pass along the strategies that my clients and I have used to achieve maximum (i.e. age-group world-qualifying) performance in fewer hours. I've worked with high-power executives, graduate students, intercontinental pilots and time-strapped parents, all of whom have been able to achieve lofty performance goals without decaying into ego-centric, self-obsessed triathletes. If you wish to be fast as well as capable of discussing something besides training at dinner parties, this book is for you.

What I am assuming you want to achieve

The framework and principles of the Working Triathlete are informed by the assumption that you are motivated to perform well. Though you could haphazardly exercise each day at a random pace and still finish a triathlon, I am assuming that you want to reach your maximum potential given your time constraints. To do this, you need a sustainable and well-structured plan that aligns with your lifestyle and allows you to achieve performance gains in the most brutally efficient manner possible. This does not mean that all training prescribed herein will be painless or effortless, but it will be balanced, time-efficient and fulfilling. Whether you travel for work half the week, are in the throes of medical residency, or put in the typical 9-5, you can achieve great results if you glean recommendations from this book and assimilate them into your training.

What this book is not

Although beginners will reap value from reading this book and adhering to its principles, my focus is on conveying an approach that committed athletes can harness to get faster. This is not a "My First Mini Triathlon" kind of book, nor is it driven by a "Just Finish" philosophy. Certainly not everyone can or should be gunning for the podium, but there is much satisfaction to be gained from setting challenging performance goals and achieving them — whatever they may be. As such, the intent of this book is not to be a comprehensive primer on all things triathlon or serve as a shortcut to the finish line; the intent it is to convey a concentrated approach that dedicated athletes (beginners and elites alike) can use to boost race performance.

How this book is structured

The first part of this book (Chapters 1-4) covers the more technical aspects of training, including the training cycle, zones and other nitty gritty items. After laying out the foundational vocabulary, I explain how the Working Triathlete approach differs from other plans and what a typical macrocycle looks like. In Chapter 5, I go over the special principles that drive an efficient training program, including hacks and tips that will get you fitter faster.

In the second part of the book, I dive into the disciplines and explore each the swim, bike and run in more detail and explain how each fits into the training plan. I also cover the importance of strength training and offer core exercises that you can utilize to efficiently build power and remain durable.

The third part of the books contains two training plans: one 12-week General Prep plan and one 12-week half iron plan. Utilize these to see how a macrocycle evolves and as a framework for your own training. More detailed plans are available at www.workingtriathete.com.

Throughout the book we will discuss the training approaches of four real-world athletes to see how each, with their unique schedules, backgrounds and abilities, were able to successfully train for and exceed their goals.

Why this books is unique

There is no shortage of triathlon books and training plans available for sale and many will make you faster. However, most come from a general and inoffensive perspective as they try to cater to the masses. They lack a niche focus and tend to be filled with a lot of fluff trying to be all things to all athletes. If you have not guessed it yet, Working Triathlete, although grounded in proven training principles, does not take the traditional approach to training. The purpose here is not to repackage the common textbook knowledge pervading triathlon into a riskless philosophy, relate it to a boiler plate training regimen and have athletes execute it. Rather, the purpose is to equip you with knowledge derived from sound training principles that will allow you to adapt the hyper-focused training plans herein in an efficient manner to suit your lifestyle. The goal is to make you ruthlessly and unapologetically efficient so that you can perform (and excel) in not only triathlon, but in all areas of your life.

Contents

Chapter 1

Types of Time-Strapped Triathletes

Training is not one size fits all

Errrr, errrr, errrr! The alarm clock wails as Maximus rubs his eyes. He can hardly believe that it is already 4:00 AM. After verifying that he did not accidentally move the clock forward five hours before going to sleep, he accepts the unbelievable reality: it is, in fact, time to wake up. He lets out a long sigh and a choice four letter word, questioning his decision to train for an iron distance race. One would think that two decades of 5AM swim practices would have made it easy for him to pop out of bed; but his ability to adapt does not extend to waking up early. As a young sales professional in NYC, he has grown accustomed to long work days and happy hours, but morphing into an early bird remains a struggle. The training plan that he downloaded from the internet calls for 17 hour training weeks, so he has conceded miserably to waking up before the sun rises to pack in the volume. As he stumbles to his closet to find a clean pair of running shorts, he wonders if there is a way to be competitive and not wake up before the rooster crows.

Meanwhile across town, Kim is already in the kitchen brewing her morning espresso shot. The mom and corporate executive cherishes her mornings since they are the only time she can be alone with her thoughts. She views her morning workout routine as a way to meditate, reset and recharge. Waking up is easy, but she is looking to spice up her training and complete a half iron distance race within a year. Since evenings are reserved for spending time with her family, she is wondering if she has the bandwith to appropriately train.

Different lifestyles, similar approach

Though Maximus and Kim have different schedules, different motivating factors for doing triathlons, and different strengths and weaknesses, their needs are similar: to train efficiently without sacrificing performance or compromising other pursuits. Over the years, I have worked with athletes who have horrifying schedules, strong and weak backgrounds in all or none of the sports, and both selfish and charitable reasons for racing. However, in most of these instances, it was possible to achieve remarkable results by adhering to universal training philosophies while making intelligent adjustments unique to individual situations.

In this chapter, I want to present four real-life athletes (you already know Maximus and Kim) with varying backgrounds and schedules. You may see yourself in one or all of these athletes, but each should hopefully provide some useful takeaways as you look to balance life and triathlon training. Although each of them is at a different stage in their life, they all are busy achievers with responsibilities – much like you. Despite their busy schedules, with discipline, creativity and conscientiousness each can excel in triathlon without stifling their relationships or careers.

The former collegiate athlete: Maximus the magnificent swimmer

Age: 25

Background: Maximus is a hardworking, young sales professional who lives in New York City. He is a former collegiate swimmer and is extremely competitive. He is a night owl and enjoys a bit of libations every now and then.

Training limitations: Although Maximus's competitive streak and discipline allow him to stick to a plan, he has the potential to be overly ambitious and burn out. Especially since he has little run background, it is important to build volume gradually and methodically to avoid injury.

Goal: To do an iron distance race ASAP.

Preliminary approach: It is important to rein him in and set a reasonable timeline for an adequate iron distance build. Because he is already an incredible

15

swimmer, the emphasis should be on building bike and run fitness while preserving swim ability and confidence. He has tremendous natural talent and wants to perform well, so it is important to press the envelope in training while still ensuring that he remains healthy. Since he rarely crawls into bed before midnight, most key sessions should be in the afternoons or evenings.

The time-strapped, high powered CFO: Kim the corporate exec

Age: 42

Background: Kim is a CFO at an investment firm and is married with two children. She works long hours and her job is stressful, but she loves it. She tries to work out five or six times per week, with four or five of these sessions being runs. She is health conscious and has completed one sprint triathlon, albeit slowly. She does have some experience in all three sports.

Training limitations: Because of her life responsibilities, Kim can only work out once per day in the morning. Her workload increases dramatically around quarter end.

Goal: To complete a half iron race within a year.

Preliminary approach: By necessity, Kim is going to have a steady diet of morning brick workouts. Although not ideal, a well-structured plan composed of weekday bricks and good endurance sessions on the weekends is the best approach. The toughest challenge will be balancing training with a high-stress job and family.

The older, busy, uber-biker: Bill the biker

Age: 59

Background: Bill is a consultant based out of San Francisco who travels 2-3 days per week. He is married with three mostly grown children. As an avid cyclist, he has a strong aerobic engine. He has very little run experience apart from hopping in a few local 5Ks, but the swim is his biggest weakness. He can barely doggy paddle two laps in a 25-yard pool and he has a subtle but genuine fear of drowning.

Training limitations: Bill's travel schedule often causes him to forgo working out, leading to inconsistent training during the week. As an older athlete, he is more injury prone.

Goal: Bill wants to become competitive in local triathlons, build general fitness and be healthy.

Preliminary approach: Bill needs to focus on two things above all else: getting comfortable in the water and preventing injury. These can be achieved through joining a Masters Swim group, building volume gradually and adhering to a good strength routine.

The creative free spirit who can't really bike: Imogene the artist

Age: 30

Background: Imogene is a freelance graphic artist who enjoys the hip, somewhat nomadic lifestyle. She also places a high priority on volunteering and is a board member at two local charity organizations focused on helping underprivileged youth. She enjoys working out, but it has mostly been limited to yoga and Pilates. She took swim lessons as a child and runs once or twice a week, but she has never done any serious road cycling apart from a casual ride on the greenway. She has recently taken up mountain biking, but her lack of cycling strength is inhibiting her ability to ride on basic trails. Don't let her calm and cool exterior fool you, she has ferocious focus and is a very hard worker.

Training limitations: Imogene has a limited sports background and is not particularly interested in tracking training data. She works a lot and has a rich social life that she wishes to preserve.

Goal: She wants to do local shorter races and build up to an off-road triathlon or half iron race.

Preliminary approach: The key for Imogene is creating and adhering to a simple and efficient plan. The initial emphasis should be on building bike fitness and keeping workouts short.

Tailoring the training plan

Throughout this book you will see these four athletes pop up in various chapters as we address their special circumstances and develop solutions that will allow them to maximize the effectiveness of their training with minimal time investment.

Each of these athletes possesses unique goals and lifestyles. There are, however, certain fundamental commonalities between them, most notably the necessity to approach training with efficiency. Because they all have demanding jobs and people who rely on them, they cannot afford to engage in a self-absorbed training regimen composed of hours upon hours of aerobic exercise. Nevertheless, they have ambitious goals and the desire to chase them. These are the kinds of athletes for whom Working Triathlete was created, so let us bust the concept that one has to be an absent parent, distant spouse or distracted worker to race exceptionally well.

Chapter 2

Low Volume Philosophy

The rationale driving the Working Triathlete

Volume is not everything...efficiency, consistency, adaptability and specificity are

Unlike what you have heard from your hardcore triathlon friends or read in articles covering professionals, you do not need to commit an inordinate amount of time to training in order to progress and become accomplished. Volume is just one tiny component of training and there have been countless examples of individuals (e.g. Kim, Maximus, Bill and Imogene) performing remarkably well by training ~6-12 hours per week or less over a training cycle and beating athletes who brag about slogging through 20+ hour weeks. What separates the individuals who perform well off of a limited time commitment from those who spend all day training with minimal payoff is not usually genetics – it is an understanding of the precise stimulus the body requires to get faster and the efficient execution of key workouts on a consistent basis to achieve steady and relentless progress. These athletes do what they need to do to get faster and nothing else.

The overarching philosophy in the Working Triathlete is that frequent and specific stimulus at key intensities throughout the training cycle can be achieved in a flexible, time efficient manner that will allow typical or exceptional athletes to approach their genetic potential.

Beyond a modest point, fitness gains become incremental. Although incremental gains are still gains, for a working triathlete striving for efficiency, the rewards of obsessing over hitting an arbitrary volume goal are not worth the costs — whether the costs are time, money, psychological fatigue or a frustrated family. For example, there may be a marginal benefit to disappearing into your pain cave and doing a weekly four-hour indoor bike ride in winter six months before your A-race. Who knows, maybe you need a break from your kids and dog and a half day of being alone in your guest bedroom pedaling is actually an appealing proposition. If that's the case, go for it. But from a fitness perspective, a better return on investment would be engaging in shorter, higher intensity workouts that efficiently boost strength, power and aerobic capacity. The idea is that by intelligently designing your training plan, you can gain all or nearly all the benefits of high-cost training by strategically replacing these sessions with low-cost, high-benefit sessions, in pursuit of becoming a complete athlete.

Low-Cost, High Benefit Training

All workouts are not created equally. To truly maximize the benefits of training and achieve more in fewer hours, you must prioritize the execution of certain workouts over others and understand the relative value and cost of various sessions. To do this, you should emphasize workouts that deliver maximum benefit with minimal cost. This should be the goal of any training plan: strike the appropriate balance between your workouts' costs and benefits and position those workouts appropriately within the larger training cycle, and you can get faster in less time and with less overall physical and mental stress.

What is the cost of a workout?

Every workout has a cost, the most obvious of which is time investment. For most working professionals, squeezing in workouts around a busy life is going to be the most difficult training variable. For example, Kim the corporate exec must fit in her weekday training sessions before work, so long weekday workouts are not feasible, nor are two-a-days. But there are other considerations as well, such as how exhausting a workout is and how much psychological and physical stress it causes. For Maximus the magnificent swimmer, his struggles waking up in the morning might not be worth the mental anguish if he can fit in training over his lunch break or in the evening. For sake of simplicity, you can distill a workout's cost into the acronym DPPR, which stands for duration, physical impact, psychological impact and recovery requirements

-**Duration**, or the overall time commitment a workout requires (including prep and travel time). The higher the duration, the less time you have for other pursuits. This is usually the most important cost component for time-strapped triathletes.

-**Physical Impact**, or how tiring the workout is physically. Imogene the artist, for example, would likely have little energy to commit to volunteering if her training load was excessive, so striving for a realistic and balanced plan is imperative.

-**Psychological Impact**, or how stressful the workout is mentally, including stress accrued before, during and after the workout. Bill the uber biker's fear of swimming might lead him to dread his swim workouts, so the psychological impact from swim sessions (at least at first) would be greater for him than others. Keeping the workouts short, targeted and perhaps social, might alleviate some of his dread.

-**Recovery Costs**, or how much time and effort is required to adequately recover from a workout. Bill and Maximus, both of whom travel a lot and interact with people, may become burnt out or sick due to an inability to adequately recover between workouts, leading to a potentially compromised immune system and dysfunctional endocrine system. Remember that recovery is as important as the training itself.

Lowering your workouts' costs enable you to be more consistent

Believe it or not, willpower, motivation and discipline are limited resources. Although you can strengthen and develop these traits, at a certain point, you are going to burn out. More than anything, what is going to allow you to gain fitness is the persistent execution of workouts over successive days, weeks and months. To achieve the kind of steady, long-term consistency required to maximize fitness and still perform in other areas of your life, you need to leverage your limited psychological resources in the most economical manner possible.

Variation between individuals

Just because a workout is high-cost for one person does not mean it is high-cost for another. Your own individual wiring may influence which factors increase a workout's cost and you should honestly assess which workouts are most troublesome. If you're like Maximus, you may dread waking up at 4:30 AM for the early Masters Swim practice, but you do it every weekday anyway because someone told you it's what great swimmers do. Because you drag yourself out of bed so early, you generally hate the practices, are half-asleep for most of them and are only getting five hours of sleep each night. You are, in fact, burning yourself out. A solution may be moving your schedule around to fit in afternoon or evening practices with the team, or cutting back to three sessions per week and making them count. This way, the costs — sleep deprivation, psychological stress, negative impact on other workouts, etc. — are minimized, leaving you fresh for your other training sessions and life responsibilities. Be honest with yourself and recognize that balance breeds consistency.

But remember, getting faster isn't free

This is not to say that all workouts you execute can or should be low-cost. There is no way around it: to prepare well for the rigors of racing, you need to put in time and effort. Racing fast requires tremendous physical and mental fortitude and you must get comfortable stimulating and strengthening the physiological and psychological systems that you will need to tap into during races. To do this, you need to stress these systems in training, which often does not feel good in the moment. Some days Maximus is going to have go wake up early, Imogene is going to be sore from a tough cycling workout and Bill is going to be nauseous from the perpetual smell of chlorine in his nostrils. The overarching goal, however, should be to achieve the desired stimuli, or maximum benefit, in the most efficient — i.e., low-cost — manner possible

How to maximize the benefit of your training

To get faster in fewer hours, you need to focus on executing an appropriately balanced mix of high-benefit workouts throughout the training cycle. The purpose of every training session is to generate specific physiological responses so that the body can adapt and become fitter. The extent to which the body adapts to a given workout or series of workouts is its benefit. If you want to maximize efficiency, you need to maximize the benefit of your workouts while minimizing costs. To do this, you need to strategically execute a diverse combination of the workouts, including general endurance, threshold, VO2/aerobic capacity and long endurance sessions (see the Nitty Gritty chapter for more information on workout types).

Most training plans prescribe a mix of these workouts at some point in the training cycle. The problem, however, comes in the way the various workouts are integrated into the schedule. While it might look good on paper, doing a long ride on Saturday, a long run on Sunday and multiple high-duration supporting sessions each week for months on end — which is what many plans prescribe — it might not be psychologically or physiologically sustainable for a working athlete. Simply throwing volume at athletes can lead to good results if they don't break, but it's a misguided approach for individuals who are time-strapped. Most training plans, in an effort to appear balanced, check all the boxes and contain all the buzz words, integrate too much volume (duration+frequency) which leads to excess load (intensity+volume) that is detrimental, or at the very least not beneficial, to the athlete. The truth is, so long as consistency/frequency is emphasized and the correct balance of intensity is implemented at appropriate times, you can make remarkable gains in triathlon fitness on less volume (i.e. in less time) than you might realize.

Upping your intensity

In most cases, your body gains fitness faster and more effectively with higher-intensity sessions, so the benefit is usually greater. There is a massive amount of nuance in that statement and many athletes/coaches will inevitably misinterpret it and blow up my inbox with messages challenging its veracity, so I do need to clarify what I mean. I want to emphasize right off the bat that Zone 2 general endurance sessions still need to compose the bulk of your training; however, the science backing the effectiveness of high-intensity work is irrefutable, especially if you do not have the time to put in a massive amount of volume during the early Preparation Phase of your training cycle (i.e., you aren't a professional athlete with the luxury of engaging in and recovering from 25-35 hours of Z1-2 work each week). If you are looking to maximize fitness gains in the most efficient manner possible, you need to intelligently execute a sizeable percentage of your training at a higher intensity while still nurturing your base aerobic fitness and recovering adequately.

The Working Triathlete, however, is not a high-intensity training regimen

Nearly everyone has heard of the outsized benefits of high-intensity interval training (HIIT), the actual definition of which may vary, but for our purposes I will classify "high intensity," (HIT or HIIT) as intervals in upper-Zone 3 to Zone 5. The concept that performing intervals at high intensities leads to superior fitness gains has been heralded in recent years — and for good reason. There are dozens of studies that support the effectiveness of high intensity training and its relative superiority over traditional, low-intensity endurance training at leading to various physiological adaptations including increased heart stroke volume, skeletal muscle oxidative capacity, muscle enzyme levels, anaerobic threshold, VO2 max and exercise economy (Burgomaster 2008; Costill 1988; Daussin 2008; Helgerud 2007; Londeree 1997; Weston 1997).

It is clear that the body adapts incredibly well to bouts of HIT and, in a perfect world, you would just train at a high intensity each day to achieve enormous fitness gains. Unfortunately, due to the cost of high-intensity workouts, this is not feasible. Too many low-volume plans take the approach of throwing out supporting sessions and neglecting base mileage in favor of unremitting hard sessions. They call for fewer overall sessions each week, but they require that all of them be intense. The problem with this approach is that athletes often plateau, get injured or end up dreading their workouts and burning out.

On the other side of the spectrum, many traditional approaches misconstrue the general concept of periodization and place too much emphasis on Zone 1 and 2 training throughout the macrocycle. Often, these plans take periodization to mean that all training during the base or Preparation Phase should be at low intensities, so the prescription ends up being easy aerobic sessions for half a macrocycle or more. This causes athletes to lose touch with the neural and muscular demands of higher-intensity efforts and, more importantly, miss out on the wonderful and efficient cardiorespiratory benefits of such sessions. Although overall training load should be lower early in the training cycle compared to later on, high-intensity sessions can and should be integrated intelligently — i.e., with adequate recovery and with volume appropriate for their placement within the macrocyle.

Relative to traditional plans, a truly effective time-efficient approach to training like the one described in this book requires a greater percentage of working time to be spent at higher intensities. The benefits are tremendous relative to the time invested. However, it is essential that their timing and format fit strategically into the overall framework of the training plan so that the athlete can gain fitness, adequately recover, avoid burnout and peak at the appropriate time.

The approach of Working Triathlete is not to just add HIT days. It is to create a framework for training that is informed by irrefutable principles that maximize efficiency, recovery and effectiveness throughout the training cycle.

Chapter 3

The Nitty Gritty: Training Zones and other Jargon

Clarifying concepts so that you know what I'm talking about

Triathlon training can get as complicated as you want it to be. Many love geeking out over data and metrics, while others despise it. Fortunately, you do not need a degree in statistics to become a great triathlete. To maximize efficiency, though, you need a fundamental understanding of training concepts and the purposes behind certain workouts — even if, like Imogene, you hate wearing a watch.

Regardless of your level of knowledge, I encourage you to read this chapter closely (it might be dense for some, but plow on). Sometimes there is variation between one training philosophy's definitions of certain words or concepts and others', and I want to remove any ambiguity up front and clarify precisely what I mean when I refer to specific terms and ideas. When you are looking to wring every drop of potential from your training, it is essential that you execute workouts at prescribed intensities and understand their intent.

Intensity Zones

Intensity zones refer to the level of intensity you should be exerting at any given time within a workout. For most of the purposes within the Working Triathlete, there will be five intensity zones, with Zone 1 being the easiest and Zone 5 being an effort near your VO2 max (i.e. the highest rate at which your body can deliver oxygen to your muscles and produce energy aerobically). The main zones key off of a metric, such as a percentage of a target heart rate measured in beats per minute (BPM) or some pace/power that you determine via a field test or race. If you cannot measure your heart rate, speed, or power, you can also key off of a level of

26

perceived exertion on a 1-10 scale, often referred to as rated perceived exertion (RPE), with 1-2 being extremely easy (Zone 1 — you can sing), 3-4 being easy (Zone 2 — you can easily speak in full sentences), 5-6 being moderate to somewhat hard (Zone 3 — you are getting winded speaking), 7-8 being moderately hard (Zone 4 — you probably do not feel like talking) and 9-10 being hard (Zone 5 — no talking; think of race pace for events lasting ~4-15 minutes).

Determining Intensity Zones: the importance of establishing your thresholds

For our purposes, your threshold for the bike and run refers to the highest intensity you are capable of exerting for an hour and is smack dab in the middle of Zone 4. For the swim, it is around the pace you can swim for a 1000 meter time trial. It is important to know your threshold pace, power and/or heart rate for each the swim, bike and run because the other zones are calculated relative to them. For example, Zone 2 on the bike is stipulated as 69-83% of your cycling threshold heart rate, or 56-75% of your functional threshold power; and Zone 2 of the swim is your threshold pace plus 10 seconds. To establish your threshold, I recommend performing threshold field tests and monitoring your heart rate and pace/power during these tests in order to define your threshold heart rate (THR), functional threshold power (FTP) and/or threshold pace.

Note: Many plans prescribe intensity zones off of a percentage of maximum heart rate. Although this can work, it is extremely difficult and exhausting to measure maximum heart rate and the common formula (i.e., 220 minus your age) is worthless as there is tremendous variation among individuals. For these reasons, I recommend utilizing the threshold calculation method.

How to establish your threshold for each discipline

There are various methods you can use to establish your threshold power/pace or heart rate for each the swim, bike and run. The easiest way is via field tests within each discipline wherein you exert a maximum effort for a certain period of time and harness the results to extrapolate a threshold metric. Following are brief explanations of what I consider the best field tests for each discipline.

Cycling: 20-minute test to establish functional threshold power (FTP)

Simply warm up for approximately 20-30 minutes and perform a five-minute interval close to an all-out effort. After a five minute recovery, ride as hard as you can for 20 minutes, tracking your average power over this 20-minute effort. By the end, you should be seeing stars. Take that average power and subtract 5%. This is your FTP. On a different day, ride at your FTP for 15-20 minutes. Your heart will stabilize at your threshold heart rate (THR).

If you don't have a power meter but want to establish your threshold heart rate, warm up for 15-20 minutes and then ride an all-out, 30-minute time trial by yourself while tracking your heart rate. Your average heart rate over the final 20 minutes of the time trial is your THR.

Running: 30-minute field test to establish threshold running pace

Warm up for 15 minutes and perform drills and strides. Run a 30-minute, all-out time trial by yourself on a track or other measurable course. Your average pace over the 30-minute time trial is your threshold pace and your average heart rate over the last 20 minutes of the effort is your threshold heart rate. Remember, run HARD.

Swimming: 1000-y/m time trial to establish threshold or T-Pace

Swim 1000 meters or yards as fast as you can. Your average pace per 100 is your threshold pace or T-Pace. If you are a beginner or have difficulty swimming 1000 yards or meters, you can swim 3X300 y/m with 30 seconds of rest. Your average pace per 100 is your T-Pace.

Intensity Zones for Swim, Bike and Run

Following are metrics showing how the various intensity zones relate to your threshold pace and HR for each discipline:

Training Intensity Zones

Zone 1

RPE: 1 to 2 **Purpose:** Active Recovery

Swim pace per 100: Easy or technique

Bike % FTP: <55% **Bike % THR:** <69%

Run Pace: Very Easy **Run % THR:** <85%

Zone 2

RPE: 3-4 **Purpose:** Endurance

Swim pace per 100: T-Pace plus 10 seconds

Bike % FTP: 56-75% **Bike % THR**: 69-83%

Run Pace: Easy **Run % THR:** 85-89%

Zone 3

RPE: 5-6 **Purpose:** Tempo

Swim pace per 100: T-Pace plus 5 seconds

Bike % FTP: 76-90% **Bike % THR**: 84-94%

Run Pace: Moderate **Run % THR:** 85-89%

Zone 4

RPE: 7-8 **Purpose:** Threshold

Swim pace per 100: T-Pace

Bike % FTP: 91-105% **Bike % THR:** 95-105%

Run Pace: Half Marathon to 10K **Run % THR:** 95-99%

Zone 5

RPE: 9-10 **Purpose:** VO2 Max

Swim pace per 100: T-Pace minus 5 seconds

Bike % FTP: 106-120% **Bike % THR:** >105%

Run Pace: 3K-5K **Run % THR:** >100%

What These Zones Accomplish: Types of Workouts

Any good training plan will have a mix of workouts that emphasize certain intensity zones. This is because different intensities lead to physiological adaptations unique to that zone. For sake of simplicity, you can conceptualize these zones applying to four main workout types: general endurance work, threshold work, VO2 work and long endurance sessions.

General Aerobic Conditioning/Endurance Work (Zones 1-3): refers to low-intensity "base" work or supporting sessions; think of easy or steady runs, manageable bike rides and moderate, form-focused swims. Most of your training time should be in these lower zones as it carries little recovery cost while effectively leading to an increase in mitochondrial enzymes, fat utilization, lactate clearance and general aerobic capacity/cardiorespiratory function. Zone 1 and 2 should feel quite easy, and Zone 3 should begin feeling moderately hard—more of a tempo effort.

Threshold Work (Zone 4): refers to harder, focused efforts, usually in the form of intervals; think of 10K to half-marathon intensity, 1000-yard swim race pace or the maximum pace you can sustain on a bike for an hour. This effort is approximately that at which your body reaches the limit of its ability to efficiently clear lactate from the bloodstream. As the name implies, it is particularly effective at boosting your lactate threshold.

VO2 or High Intensity Interval Work (Zone 5): refers to intense efforts usually in the form of short (<8 minutes) intervals; think of hard swim intervals, 800-meter track intervals at 5K pace, or leg-busting 6x4 minute intervals on the bike. The pace is intense and can lead to similar adaptations as with lower intensity work, but to a greater extent and with the outsized benefit of dramatically increasing cardiac output and oxygen utilization.

Long Rides/Runs (Usually Zone 2 -3): refer to key endurance sessions that are substantially longer than other workouts and which utilize most of your glycogen stores. These sessions lead to important metabolic, muscular and cardiovascular adaptations that occur beyond certain duration. Long workouts teach you to withstand the fatigue that results from prolonged bouts of exercise and enable you to burn more fat as fuel. They also serve a great practice purpose, allowing you to hone in on the best nutrition and pacing strategies for longer races. Although beneficial and necessary, these workouts come at high recovery costs.

These four classifications fail to capture the nature of all workouts. For example, there are strength-building sessions (i.e., low-cadence work on the bike and hill running), hybrid sessions and workouts unrelated to endurance (i.e., weight training), though the core of any good endurance regimen is predominately composed of the above four types.

Key and Supporting Sessions

Beyond understanding the general types of workouts, you should be aware of the importance of certain workouts relative to others. Sessions that take priority within a week or microcycle are referred to as key sessions, whereas others, although important, are referred to as supporting sessions.

Key Sessions

Classified as either key intensity or key endurance, key sessions are the most essential workouts on the schedule. If you are time-strapped, you should prioritize the execution of these since they are most indispensable for efficiently gaining fitness. For example, if Kim the corporate executive has a 6 AM flight to catch for a day trip to Chicago and hence only 35 minutes for a workout (since she is taking her children to a theater production later that night), she should strive to structure her weekly schedule so that a supporting session falls on her travel day. Ideally, the most important key sessions should be performed on days when you have the ability to commit the appropriate amount of time and energy to them.

Usually, you will have one key intensity session and one key endurance session within each discipline each week. Though the overall load of these sessions vary, typical key intensity sessions are composed of tempo/threshold or VO2 efforts, whereas key endurance sessions are your longer efforts (e.g., long ride, run and swim). By elevating the importance of key sessions, you ensure that your body receives the most beneficial, well-rounded stimulus for developing fitness.

Supporting Sessions

Supporting sessions, although of secondary importance to key sessions, are absolutely necessary for maintaining and building endurance. These are commonly of lower duration and intensity than the key sessions, though their frequency allows you to build basic cardiorespiratory fitness as well as the durability required to successfully complete key sessions. The ideal plan maximizes the load of supporting sessions while still ensuring adequate recovery and freshness necessary for nailing the key sessions.

We all know that life happens and sometimes we have to be creative and adapt. When working with Imogene the artist, it was clear that she despised cycling indoors by herself. She, like many people, preferred spin classes, mountain biking, or leisurely cycling on greenways. But she also loved having time to commit to her own art and volunteer work and also wanted to get faster. Because of this, we eliminated supporting cycling sessions that occurred indoors on her trainer, and instead ensured that every indoor session was a key session that she could accomplish efficiently, or alternatively, was a group spin class. However, we were careful not to diminish the importance of supporting sessions, so whenever the weather was nice outside (something rare in rainy Seattle), we would adapt the plan to take advantage of her new-found love of outdoor cycling by strategically scheduling supporting or long cycling sessions outdoors. Although being flexible in this manner required extra work and creative planning, it enhanced her enjoyment of training, prevented burnout and allowed her to gain fitness while minimizing cost.

By understanding workout types and adhering to stipulated intensity zones, you will be able to execute your sessions more efficiently and reap greater fitness gains from the work you do. Training is about balancing load with recovery, the former of which is very much governed by the intensity you exert. By hitting the correct intensities for the correct duration relative to your fitness level and prioritizing certain workouts, you will maximize fitness gains and ensure that every minute of training has a purpose.

Chapter 4

The Training Cycle

Getting fast requires knowing how to train

Now that we have established basic training concepts and Working Triathlete-specific philosophy, we should zoom out to better understand periodization, the larger macro training cycle and, most importantly, how Working Triathlete differentiates itself from the traditional approach.

This chapter, like the Nitty Gritty chapter, is dense, but important. Understanding it is how you get fast. So press on. Subsequent chapters will be much more captivating.

Periodization

The basic idea of periodization is to structure a training cycle so that an athlete's fitness peaks for a specific competition. All training within a training cycle is structured so as to maximize physical preparedness for a single race or narrow sequence of races. The Working Triathlete training model adheres to the general concept of periodization, though it strays from the traditional model in certain respects to account for decreased volume. You will find the same phases in the traditional model — Preparation, Competition and Transition (further discussed in this chapter) — though the specific nature of workouts and their intensities will deviate.

The Parts of the Training Plan

There are three main components within a training cycle which serve as descriptors when referring to certain time periods within the plan. These are the macrocycle, mesocycle and microcycle.

Macrocycle

The macrocycle, which very often encompasses a full season or year, refers to the overarching training plan building to a specific race. The macrocycle is broken down into three main phases: the Preparation Phase, the Competition Phase and the Transition Phase.

Mesocycle

A mesocycle refers to a time block of training within the macrocycle. It typically lasts 2-8 weeks and is defined by the specific training focus the block emphasizes, such as aerobic fitness, aerobic capacity, strength, technique/tactics, etc.

Microcycle

A microcycle is an even smaller training block, usually lasting a week. Conceptually, the microcycle serves to segregate a series of workouts into a particular cadence and position within a mesocycle and macrocycle. Because it makes sense conceptually and practically, microcycles are usually Monday to Sunday, allowing an athlete and coach to focus on the execution of workouts on a more basic and immediate level.

Phases of a Macrocycle

What defines the periodization model of training is the deconstruction of the training plan into Phases, each of which emphasizes certain training goals. The three main phases are the Preparation, Competition and Transition Phases, which can further be broken down into Subphases.

Preparation Phase

The Preparation Phase, the earlier part of which is sometimes referred to as the Base Phase, is the longest and most important Phase. Especially in the early Preparation Phase, there is traditionally a lot of low-intensity work that lays the basic foundation of aerobic fitness upon which higher intensity training is built. The Phase can be broken down into two Subphases: the General Preparation Subphase, which is largely composed of general endurance building, and the Specific

Preparation Subphase, which more thoroughly integrates race-specific intensities such that training load reaches (or, at the very least, approaches) its highest point. The Preparation Phase typically lasts 8-16 weeks, though it can span a much longer (or shorter) timeframe depending on the individual and his/her schedule.

Competition Phase

The next phase is the Competition Phase, which occurs directly after the Preparation Phase. This phase is broken down further into the Pre-Competition and Competition Subphases. The Pre-Competition Subphase is an extension of the Specific Preparation Subphase in that training load is still high, but there is an even more fervent emphasis on race preparation. As the Competition Phase progresses beyond the Pre-Competition Subphase and into the Competition Subphase, there is a continued focus on race readiness as volume decreases and intensity remains high. Depending on the schedule, this Subphase may contain numerous races, with the priority race typically occurring at the end of the Competition Subphase. Taken as a whole, the Competition Phase is usually shorter than the Preparation Phase, lasting 6-10+ weeks, though the actual duration can vary.

Transition Phase

The third and final phase is the Transition Phase, which is a period of little to no training between macrocycles that allows the mind and body to recover and recharge. This phase may contain active recovery, non-triathlon related activities or complete rest. The idea is to reset physically and mentally so that you can begin the next macrocycle refreshed and focused.

Base, Build, Taper Concepts

In addition to the Phase/Subphase concept, you might have heard of other blocks within a training plan, specifically Base, Build and Taper Periods. These are useful in describing how the training load (volume+intensity) varies throughout the macrocycle. Conceptually, you should envision the Base Period encompassing most of the Preparation Phase as training load gradually increases. The Build Period represents the period within the macrocycle when load is at its highest, which occurs during the latter part of the Preparation Phase into the Pre-Competition Subphase. After the Build Period, you enter your Taper, which is a reduction in load to alleviate fatigue and sharpen fitness for the goal race.

Below is a chart visually outlining the Phases of a macrocycle, as well as the Base, Build and Taper Periods:

Macrocycle				
10-24+ weeks				
Preparation Phase (Base Phase) 5-16+ weeks		Competition Phase 6-10+weeks		Transition Phase 2-8 weeks
Base	Build	Taper	Race	Rest

Why periodization works

The periodization model of training has been around for decades and has proven to lead to stellar performance. The main reason it has endured so long and remains, for the most part, legitimate, is because the body cannot maintain a high training load over the long term. Eventually, your body, mind and fitness break down, hence the value of a cycle of recovery and rebuilding. Additionally, the periodization model allows for gradual and comprehensive adaptation to training volume, meaning that the early Preparation Phase prepares the athlete's bones, tendons and joints to withstand an increasing training and racing load throughout the Competition Phase.

How the Working Triathlete framework differs

Although the traditional model of executing mostly low-intensity training throughout the Preparation Phase (which can last 2/3-3/4 of the duration of a macrocycle) can boost fitness and durability, many coaches and athletes have the propensity to oversimplify and schedule only easy aerobic work during this Phase. This approach is alarmingly inefficient — especially for an athlete who never intends to crank out massive 25-35-hour weeks. For low-volume athletes, there is no reason to completely eliminate higher-intensity efforts, even in the earliest stages of the Preparation Phase. To do so would mean to needlessly discard fitness benefits in an effort to adhere to a training philosophy intended for high-volume athletes.

This is not to say that training should look the same throughout the macrocycle or that the intensity of the General Preparation Subphase should match the Specific Preparation Subphase. It should not. However, whereas many plans stipulate that all efforts within the early Preparation Phase should be in the Zone 2 range, a low-volume working triathlete is best served executing consistent workouts — even during the General Preparation Phase — in the upper Zone 3 and lower Zone 4 range. This does not mean that you should be spending an hour in Zone 4 every day throughout the winter or early Preparation Phase; however, you should not shy away from executing solid tempo and threshold work, or even the occasional short VO2 workout. Your overall intensity during the early Preparation Phase should not be as high as it is in the Specific Prep or Competition Phases of training; however, assuming you are looking to maximize performance on fewer hours throughout the whole macrocycle, you should certainly be executing a mix of workouts in Zones 3-5 during all Phases (with the exception of the Transition Phase).

A glimpse into the specifics of a Working Triathlete macrocycle

Although the general trajectory of the Working Triathlete mirrors the traditional periodization model, there are differences. Below is a distilled explanation showing what a typical Macrocycle would look like for a triathlete under the plan.

Typical Preparation Phase (usually 8-16+ weeks)

The **General Preparation Subphase** begins with a strength-oriented mesocycle focused on functional strength endurance and aerobic work. There is a lot of low-cadence cycling, hill intervals on the run and short swim intervals. Form is emphasized and strength training, especially auxiliary movements that stabilize your joints and address muscle imbalances, are emphasized. Runs are mostly Zone 2 with brief pick-ups and strides. Rides are mostly aerobic, with some upper Z3 work and very short Zone 4/5 intervals for the neuromuscular benefit. Swim training is form based and threshold intervals are typically short, though overall swim load is comparable throughout the whole cycle. This phase of training can last quite a while (potentially multiple months) and should be scaled to fit your training calendar. You might consider it the early "base" phase of training, but light intensity should still be integrated to keep the central nervous system primed.

As the General Preparation Subphase continues and approaches the Specific Preparation Subphase, bike load increases rapidly (sooner and faster than in most training plans) with a special focus on longer Zone 3 and 4 intervals. Every single ride has some intensity, though there is sufficient recovery within and between workouts so that the body can absorb the stimulus. Run intensity remains low, with mostly Zone 2 work, though there are pick-ups in many supporting run sessions and a bit of Zone 4 work in the form of cruise intervals and tempo runs. Strides and form drills become an ever-increasingly important component of training. In the pool, longer intervals are introduced, focusing on muscular and general endurance. Strength training remains important, with a growing emphasis on developing muscular power, though it is tertiary to swimming, cycling and running.

In the **Specific Preparation Subphase**, load continues to increase. Regardless of goal race distance, long threshold intervals on the bike remain a central focus of training along with race-specific work. Run intensity remains similar to the General Preparation Subphase, though, depending on the athlete, a weekly key intensity session is usually added and frequency remains high. The duration of key endurance sessions (long rides and runs) increases, though these sessions are usually more intense and of lower duration than comparable sessions in other training plans. Swim interval length continues to increase and open water swimming and tactics are emphasized. Race-pace work becomes common and strength training remains an integral component of the plan. The overarching goal is to build high-end fitness and, as the phase continues, to spend a lot of time honing race tactics. You might consider this the build phase of training.

Typical Competition Phase (usually 6-10+ weeks)

In the **Pre-Competition Subphase,** the load that defines the Specific Preparation Subphase bleeds over, though there is a greater emphasis on race-specific work. This means that long rides and runs (if you are a long course athlete) remain important. Swim load remains high. Auxiliary strength training remains an emphasis, but power-oriented training begins to phase out.

As the **Competition Subphase** begins, intensity remains high and volume may decrease slightly, though to a lesser extent than in other training approaches. The details of the Subphase are driven by the race calendar, but as the target race draws near, there is usually a gradual two-week taper during which load decreases but intensity remains high. This unloads fatigue while still ensuring that the neuromuscular system remains primed for the demands of racing.

Typical Transition Phase (usually 2-4 weeks)

After the final race of the season, it is important to recharge and allow the body to recover from the demands of training and racing. Most should take two weeks off from triathlon training. This could mean that you do nothing or engage in active recovery. However, because the overall volume of the typical Working Triathlete macrocycle is less than other training approaches, you will not likely need to take off more than two weeks, which allows you to enter the next macrocycle sooner and more invigorated than you otherwise might have been had you adhered to a traditional, high-volume approach.

Chapter 5

The Principles

The secrets to becoming efficient

If there is only one chapter you read in the entire book, make it this one. These are the secrets that define the Working Triathlete training model.

As I mentioned, the purpose of Working Triathlete is to convey an approach that will allow you to achieve remarkable gains in as few hours of training as possible. I am not delivering a dozen different training plans tailored to every athlete's experience or specific race distance. I am delivering a framework for training and a philosophical approach that integrates strategies that allow for maximum benefit at minimum cost. By studying and attentively adhering to each of the below principles, you will transform your training and achieve significant gains in the most efficient manner possible.

#1 Frequency and consistency trump overall volume and occasional big days

If you want to get better, your primary focus should be increasing your number of sessions each week until you are running five out of seven days, cycling at least three times (four is better) and swimming at least two (three is better). Realize, however, that these workouts do not need to be separate standalone workouts, nor do they need to be long. Kim the corporate executive achieved age group podiums, including at a major 70.3, by executing brick workouts almost exclusively, with 80% of them lasting under 90 minutes. However, by engaging in two sports each day, the frequency of the stimuli made up for the lack of exceptionally long sessions. The body benefits tremendously from frequency for the following reasons:

-Specific, positive physiological adaptations occur fairly soon into the workout, so if you increase frequency, then you can decrease duration and still achieve substantial benefit — i.e., your workouts are effectively low-cost and high-benefit. To reach your potential, you need workouts of longer duration and there are certain adaptations that can only be realized with high-volume days (Kim still did a few longer weekend bricks); however, many athletes need to drop the mentality that 30-40 minute workouts are worthless. They are beneficial and can be done frequently.

-Increasing frequency is the safest and easiest way to gain fitness and increase volume to appropriate levels. Each time you work out, your body elicits an exercise-induced growth hormone response (EIGR). By increasing the frequency of your workouts, you increase the frequency of the response, thereby allowing for superior recovery and the efficient development of muscular and cardiorespiratory fitness. Additionally, by increasing the frequency of your workouts and focusing less on executing extremely long sessions, you minimize the cost of any one workout, can recover better, achieve consistency and perform key sessions at a higher intensity level. This is especially important for older athletes like Bill, who may become injured by engaging in frequent long workouts where the repetitive nature can tax certain hard and soft tissues, leading to injury or burnout.

-Apart from burning calories during exercise, working out raises your base metabolic rate for a period of time after the session is complete, often called the after-burn effect. Therefore, the more often you work out, the higher your average metabolic rate will be throughout the day, making it easier to achieve and maintain more ideal body composition for triathlon racing. This is especially important for older athletes whose metabolism has slowed down with age, but also for athletes with imbalanced diets such as Maximus, who frequents fast food places more often than he should and has a fondness for craft IPAs.

-Shorter workouts are more convenient and much easier to fit into an already busy schedule. Often, it is not necessarily that busy people do not have the time to exercise; rather, it is that they lack the large chunks of time — two to four hours — to execute workouts that they see as valuable and consistently necessary. When you focus on frequency as opposed to duration, you will find your overall weekly volume grow while the stress of trying to squeeze in long training sessions diminishes. Suddenly, the short windows of time that you thought were too brief for a workout, and which you previously wasted by spending time on Instagram or surfing Reddit, can be used for training.

Unfortunately, many athletes overlook the benefits of frequency, or feel that they need exceptionally high-volume days to be successful. Bill the uber biker had this mindset when we first began working together. As a pure cyclist, he was used to going very long. Like many athletes, he would execute the majority of his training on the weekends in the form of big sessions, thinking that shorter sessions served little purpose. Triathletes who have this mind set (i.e., those who consistently aim to execute extremely long brick workouts on the weekends) are usually rendered exhausted during the week, position themselves as likely candidates for burn out, are unable to execute and recover from beneficial high-intensity workouts, and fail to profit from frequent and consistent training. However, by elevating the importance of frequent, shorter sessions, Bill, like many of our coached athletes, saw his performance in all disciplines steadily improve. Plus he began to enjoy training more.

TLDR: Short frequent workouts are convenient, effective and essential.

#2 The 30-45, two-a-day rule

Many people view the prospect of working out two times a day as impossible or something only hardcore athletes do. These false beliefs often spring from the misunderstanding that each respective "two-a-day" workout should be hard or of equal duration to a typical "one-a-day" workout. In reality, working out twice in a day should not mean that your volume doubles — it simply means that consistency and frequency of stimulus for each of the disciplines increases. Volume does not necessarily have to increase; though, along with average intensity, volume usually does improve. Although not always possible for all athletes (e.g. Kim), by splitting the work into two shorter sessions rather than one larger one, you are fresher for a larger duration of training and can put in a superior effort with less injury risk or recovery cost.

To help athletes overcome the mental hurdle of completing two workouts and ensure they achieve frequency and consistency, I often recommend that one workout be a short 30-45 minute effort and the other a 45-60 minute effort. They do not need to be 30 and 45 minutes respectively as per the name of the rule — though that split is a good minimum target. The exact duration depends on the athlete's schedule and goal race; however, the basic concept is that one of the workouts is so short it seems like an afterthought (while still delivering a worthwhile stimulus) and can be scheduled at nearly any point in the day (hence frequent lunch time runs for Maximus), while the other "main" workout is still sufficiently short that the athlete does not dread it (so Imogene can get on her indoor trainer, knock out a targeted cycling session, and get on with her life), thereby minimizing overall cost and enabling greater consistency.

The timing of these two workouts will depend on your daily routine. I find that many athletes like to get up and knock out the shorter workout first thing in the morning because it is easy, builds momentum and does not require a wake-up call much earlier than usual to accommodate it. Other athletes who are morning people prefer to tackle the main session first. Regardless, by internalizing and habituating the concept of doing work within two different disciplines each day, you will gain technique, skill and fitness faster than you would otherwise. For most people, it is the most efficient way to maximize fitness in fewer overall hours.

I like to think of the two-a-day plan as a feasible and appeasing solution to circumvent external stress around time management, particularly when it comes to balancing training with family. Splitting your workouts into two shifts allows you to be more agile in your training: first, you can fit in your core or shorter, stimulus-inducing workout before your family awakes so that you can be present for breakfast, carpool or other family rituals. Then, you can finish your second workout (your "once you've left the office" workout) more quickly so that you can be present for a family meal, help with homework, walk the dog, etc. Obviously, we all have different life circumstances, but for those working triathletes who find themselves juggling an office life and a social/family life, it is critical to ensure that triathlon training can be weaved into that fabric and not preclude your success and happiness in other domains.

TLDR: Do two workouts each day, but keep them short so that they are manageable and more easily scheduled.

#3 If you only have time for one session each day, brick-it

Everyone's situation is different and perhaps you only have time for — or prefer — exercising a single time each day. If that is the case, brick workouts, or sessions wherein you piggyback training for two triathlon sports, are essential for maintaining frequency within each discipline (some purists might advocate that a brick workout is only a bike+run, but for our purposes we will assume it means two of any of the sports in quick succession).

Due to the benefit of specificity, it is best to do each discipline within a brick workout in the order they appear in triathlon to simulate the modularity of a race. So, for Kim, who subsisted almost entirely on brick workouts, she would usually bike before she ran and swim before anything else. However, we did not adhere stubbornly to this protocol. For example, it is decidedly uncomfortable and probably not good for the immune system to run outside in 20 degree darkness after a sweaty indoor bike session in the winter — so we would schedule the run before the bike. Executing the work in the lowest cost way trumped modularity. Don't obsess over order; just get it done.

The 30-45 rule still applies for the majority of brick workouts. Obviously, there is a time and place for longer bricks — such as a three to four-hour bike ride followed by a 20-minute run in preparation for an iron distance race — however, by keeping the majority of your bricks short and simple, especially in the preparation phase, you will be more motivated to accomplish the workouts and will not dread them, thus enabling you to gain stellar fitness in all three sports with minimized time investment. Think of sessions like a 30-minute swim chock full of intervals and a 45-minute Zone 2 run, or a 45-minute cycling session with Zone 4 intervals and a 30-minute Zone 2 run. Considering the nature of triathlon, if you only have one window of time in a day during which to work out, and that window is at least an hour, the brick is usually the superior choice, rather than devoting the entire session to a single sport.

TLDR: If you are so time-strapped that you only have one window of time each day during which to work out, choose brick workouts.

#4 You should not train like a swimmer, a runner and a cyclist. You should train like a triathlete and focus on what will make you fastest — not just faster — on race day

To maximize your potential in as few hours as possible, you need to focus on that which will make you fastest on race day. Do not view triathlon as three different sports deserving of equal focus; view it as a single sport that happens to be composed of three different disciplines. An approach wherein each discipline receives equal attention or effort is almost never the best approach. Instead, you should identify your strengths and limiters and balance your time investment in each sport so that you will improve most in areas that will save you — specifically you — the most time on race day. Maximus, for example, could break 55 minutes in an Ironman swim before he even began training with us. However, his run needed some work to be competitive, so we immediately made building his run volume a priority and lowered the number of times he swam each week from five to three. To establish your priority discipline(s), you need to do the following:

First: Know your inherent talents and ability level within each sport. Be aware of your strengths and weaknesses. Know what disciplines you are good at and what your current limiters are. Consider seeking out the counsel of an experienced coach to assist. Sometimes we are blinded by our own biases.

Second: Assess potential room for improvement within each sport. After identifying your weaknesses or limiters, assess how much time and effort would be required to improve them. If you underperform in a specific discipline, what do you have to do to get better and reach your potential? How much time are you leaving on the table by failing to address certain weaknesses? Are any of these limiters self-imposed constraints or derived from fear; can addressing a mental impasse enable improvement? Unlike Maximus, Bill, who could barely swim a lap at the start of the training cycle, needed to emphasize swim training to simply complete a sprint triathlon.

Third: Determine areas of improvement that, if addressed, would lead to the greatest potential time savings for the specific race you are training for. Take into account the proportionate duration of each discipline relative to the overall race. Attack those areas that offer the best return on invested training time. Your worst discipline may be the lowest hanging fruit, but it is also possible that the sport you are best at offers more potential time savings relative to training time investment. Your analysis should reflect your highly individualized situation.

By addressing these items, you will be able to structure a training plan that targets areas that will actually lead to improved race times — not just general fitness improvement. Everyone loves to train for their strengths, but perhaps your time would be better spent working on a neglected limiter. For example, if you are signed up for a draft legal Olympic distance race — a race in which the swim is a relatively large chunk— and you are consistently among the fastest cyclists and runners but come out of the water 10 minutes behind everyone else, it would make sense to emphasize the swim for a training cycle or two. You might add an additional session per week, get a swim coach to analyze your stroke technique, and/or schedule your swim session as the first workout of each day so that you arrive fresh and eager. One additional hour per week spent swimming, which could either be a true additional hour or reallocation of time from your cycling and running, might allow you to take five minutes off your swim with little to no detriment to your bike and run splits. This was the approach we used when working with Bill and it paid off wonderfully. Like with many first-time swimmers, he made gains much faster with a concentrated swim block and he learned to love a new sport that he can enjoy for the rest of his life.

Another situation where it makes sense to allocate a disproportionate amount of time to a specific discipline over the other two is when you are training for an iron distance race. In long course, it is difficult to overstate the importance of cycling fitness since the bike leg is, by far, the largest component of the race. You should take the swim seriously, but you should also recognize that it is a smaller portion of your day. Particularly if you are already a capable swimmer, the swimming leg is more inconsequential to your overall time than the other disciplines. The bike, however, is of sufficient duration that you cannot fake it. If you attempt to do so, it will zap your legs and render them useless for the run. Most would benefit from stressing cycling fitness over swim and run fitness, though nobody knows you as well as you. Maximus, for example, although an elite swimmer, actually took quite well to the bike and immediately showed disproportionate talent for it compared to the run. So, even though we still stressed the importance of cycling fitness during his iron distance build, we continued to prioritize the run. This approach led to massive gains in running fitness and, just as importantly, a massive increase in confidence on race day that allowed him to compete at the top of the age group field. By knowing yourself and how your abilities relate to your goal race, you can structure a training plan that will ensure superior performance

.TLDR: Structure your training so that you target areas that will make you — at an individualized level — fastest on race day.

#5 You should be aware of crossover fitness and fatigue

If you adopted the individual training philosophies of pure swimmers, cyclists and runners, you would inevitably overload on intensity and volume as you attempt to fit in multiple threshold and tough interval workouts each week in each discipline. Instead, you should be vigilant of how workouts within each sport impact the others and you should be especially aware of crossover benefit and fatigue.

Although it is true that just cycling will not make you an exceptional runner or swimmer and vice versa, there is broad aerobic crossover benefit between and among sessions that can improve fitness across disciplines. For example, you may not need to commit hours upon hours of low-intensity work building your aerobic engine on the bike if you are already experiencing aerobic crossover benefit from the volume of your run and swim sessions. Although swimming, cycling and running recruit different motor units and emphasize different muscle groups, there are general cardiorespiratory adaptations that occur within each sport that benefit all the disciplines. This is why USA Triathlon aims to recruit former collegiate runners who can swim—perhaps most notably, 2016 Olympic gold medalist Gwen Jorgenson. If you can run well, you will probably have the aerobic engine to quickly achieve a high level of cycling fitness.

Likewise, just as there is crossover benefit, there is also crossover fatigue. If you do a tough VO2 cycling workout, for example, you should avoid doing a tough VO2 run shortly thereafter due to the fatigue the former generates. It is a good practice to separate high-cost run and cycling sessions by at least 36 hours. If you execute a high-intensity workout too soon after execution of another, you may be too fatigued to commit appropriate effort to the second workout or your body may be so worn down that it cannot adequately unload the fatigue, leading to overtraining. To truly reap the benefits of efficient, higher-intensity training, make sure you provide your body appropriate time to absorb and recover from key sessions.

TLDR: Do not blindly train for the individual sports of triathlon; be aware of crossover benefit and fatigue to train more efficiently.

#6 You need a power meter and indoor trainer for your bike

This is probably the recommendation that will save you THE most amount of time while simultaneously making you fitter.

It is not negotiable.

If you want to cut the number of hours you spend in the saddle while achieving a high level of fitness, you need to invest in a power meter and indoor trainer and execute most of your cycling workouts indoors.

An indoor trainer is a tool that converts your outdoor bike into a stationary trainer. Depending on your budget, you can either purchase a simple mechanical trainer or a smart trainer. The former is cheaper and perfectly adequate in that you can adjust resistance with reasonable precision, though you have to do it manually via shifting. Smart trainers are more expensive and adjust resistance automatically and can often be synced with other technology — such as applications that simulate real-world riding — to create a more realistic indoor riding experience. From a fitness-building perspective, both types are perfectly effective so long as you actually use them.

A power meter is a device you connect to your bike — typically in the hub, pedals, bracket or crank — that measures (in watts) the amount of power you are generating while pedaling. They offer a real-time, objective measurement of your cycling performance and are useful for precisely tracking fitness and executing workouts. Once you understand how to use a power meter, you can exploit every minute on the bike and complete each interval at the appropriate intensity.

By combining a power meter with an indoor trainer, you are able to more quickly and effectively complete workouts. Relative to indoor cycling, riding outside is incredibly time consuming. It takes a lot of time getting ready to ride (helmet, GPS calibration, bike clothes, nutrition, bike check, etc.) and it often takes a while to get to an area you can ride uninhibited by traffic, stop signs and traffic lights. Having your bike always set up on an indoor trainer, however, makes it incredibly easy to knock out a cycling workout. You throw on some bike shorts, hop on, and immediately begin riding at an appropriate intensity with no interruptions or coasting. Combine this convenience with the precision of power-based training and, with the right plan, you will experience remarkable fitness gains in less time than you ever thought possible.

TLDR: Riding indoors at specific wattages is efficient and effective.

#7 You need to stop pedaling easy

Most people do not ride hard enough. For whatever reason, the concept of suffering on the bike is a foreign concept and many triathletes waste their time cruising in Zone 1or 2 for hours on end, with little to no intensity, for no exceptional fitness benefit. Perhaps it is the mentality developed from gently cycling with friends or riding as an adolescent that infects many athletes' psychologies; but the truth is, if you want to get faster on the bike, you need to spend a lot of time at a relatively high percentage of your threshold and do it consistently.

Numerous studies support the benefits of riding harder. All things being equal, high-intensity training can lead to adaptations superior to traditional steady state training. For example, a 2008 study published in The American Journal of Physiology-Regulatory, Integrative and Comparative Physiology measured the VO2 max improvements of two groups, one of which executed an 8-week HIIT cycling program with the other completing an 8-week lower intensity, continuous endurance program. Workouts were identical in duration for both groups. Subjects in the HIIT group increased their VO2 max by an average of 15% versus 9% for the steady group. According to the study, the "results suggest that fluctuations of workload and oxygen uptake during training sessions, rather than exercise duration or global energy expenditure, are key factors in improving muscle oxidative capacities. In an integrative view, IT [i.e., HIIT] seems optimal in maximizing both peripheral muscle and central cardiorespiratory adaptations, permitting significant functional improvement" (Daussin et al. 2008).

Other studies have shown that high-intensity training is superior to steady endurance training for increasing stroke volume (Helgerud et al. 2007), boosting levels of oxidative enzymes in mitochondria (Burgomaster et al. 2008) and burning fat (Boutcher 2010 and Trapp 2008).

Of course, the danger with any high-intensity program is relative cost and potential for injury. Fortunately, cycling is a comparatively low-impact sport, so you can go fairly hard on a consistent basis with little risk of injury. If most of your rides are harder (Zones 3-5), you do not need to spend inordinate amounts of time cycling, which can lower the overall cost. As previously mentioned, you are accruing a lot of aerobic training via running and swimming and do not need to put in the volume of base mileage that pure cyclists do to achieve a similar benefit. Granted, you still do need a foundation of cycling fitness and unless you are an outlier cycling should still compose the bulk of your training time. However, you should recognize that cycling prowess is most effectively and efficiently improved with higher-intensity training — sweetspot, threshold or otherwise — that can and should be done on a regular basis.

TLDR: Make your bike workouts count.

#8 Emphasize run frequency over big sessions

There is something sacred to endurance athletes about the long run. It is, in many peoples' minds, the most important workout on the schedule — a session that singularly makes one a faster runner.

This is, perhaps, the most misguided perspective in all of endurance sports.

I do not mean to demean the importance of the long run. It is a necessary component of a well-balanced training plan. However, too many athletes overemphasize its value by obsessing over it to the detriment of their other workouts. Overall run volume is more important to overall run fitness and performance than the duration of your long run. Shorter, more frequent run sessions will make you a better runner in less time and with less wear and tear on your body than longer infrequent sessions.

The long run is one of the highest-cost workouts. It stresses the joints, ligaments, muscles and bones in a more traumatic way than any other workout and is probably responsible for more overuse injuries than anything else. By dividing your weekly mileage across five or six runs, however, you can sustain higher overall volume while minimizing the likelihood of injury.

All this is not to say that you should eliminate the long run from your training regimen. If you are training for anything longer than a sprint triathlon, a good long run is absolutely essential; however, even in long course triathlon, there is no reason to run longer than two hours in training and you probably should not persistently increase the duration of your long run weekly. The benefit is infinitesimally marginal for the recovery cost. Instead, focus on running that magical 5-6 times per week before pushing your long run distance above 90 minutes and consider whether doing a long run every 10 or so days makes more sense than every seven.

TLDR: Run more often if you want to build volume in the safest and most effective way possible.

#9 Be real about the swim and make your sessions count

For many triathletes, especially those who are adult onset swimmers, the swim is an enigma. Whereas in cycling and running the harder you work the faster you go, swimming does not follow in suit. There is a tremendous technique component which, most of the time, does not come naturally for adult onset swimmers. You can have the best aerobic engine in the world, but if you are flailing in the water you will not go fast.

This reality can be frustrating for many triathletes. We all have heard of the incredibly fit 35-year-old triathlete swimming as hard as he can while a swim team of ten-year-old girls lap him in adjacent lanes. We can chalk this up to the magic of youth, but the harsh reality is that people who swam as children have a huge advantage. They likely have hundreds of thousands of yards behind them — a variable that certainly accounts for much of the discrepancy — but they also swam at a time in their lives that allowed them to develop great technique. Just as children learn languages more easily, so too do they pick up on the subtleties of the swim stroke faster than adults. They move less robotically and are able to make adjustments and fix errors in their strokes more effortlessly than adults who often stubbornly cling to their poor form.

So, what should poor swimmers do? Throw up their hands and curse that their parents did not force them to take swim lessons? Not unless you are prepared for some awkward family holidays and angsty reunions with no real impact to your swim performance itself.

With focused practice, most can achieve a decently fast swim. There are adults who, with no prior organized swim experience, are eventually able to swim under 60 minutes in an Ironman swim or even break 60 seconds for 100 yards. The commonalities among these relatively successful adult onset swimmers are a good feel for the water and sufficient adaptability to make corrections. They usually swim with others, get feedback on their technique and spend sufficient time in the pool.

If you want to reach triathlon swim greatness (a lower bar than you might think—just ask any pure swimmer) you need to swim deliberately. Hitting your local YMCA by yourself a couple times a week and mindlessly swimming laps is not going to cut it. If you want to maximize gains in fewer hours, you need to execute structured and focused workouts—ideally with others and under the watchful eye of a coach. Rare is the half-decent swimmer who does not swim with a squad or Masters group.

Nevertheless, even if an adult swimmer does all the right things, it is common to hit a plateau. Whether due to lack of coordination, swim strength or perhaps motivation to put in the required effort to get truly fast, many hit a wall and stop improving. At this point, one has to make a decision as to whether they want to invest time and energy into a massive swim block to try and get faster or to simply maintain their current ability level. Fortunately, it is fairly easy to achieve "competency" and maintain this competency with minimal time in the pool. Three times a week of focused practice, such as with a Masters Swim group, is enough frequency to see gains and two focused sessions a week is probably enough to maintain decent swim technique and fitness.

This principle is not to belittle the swim: it is important in and of itself and it also sets you up for the bike and run. Coming out of the water gassed is a recipe for disaster and if you are a poor swimmer, you need to swim more than three times per week. However, largely due to prep time, most people find swimming to be among the most time intensive of activities. You have to prepare your swimming equipment, get in the car, drive to the pool or body of water, shower, swim, shower again, change, drive home…there is a great deal of time-investment. Ideally, we would all spend time in the pool six times a week; however, when one needs to balance training within an already busy schedule, there are other sessions and other disciplines to focus on that might offer a better ROI. If you are time-strapped, focus on achieving competency and then making your swim sessions count.

TLDR: Consider the return on the hours you are investing in training. Depending on your situation, obsessing about getting in more than three focused swim sessions per week might be a poor use of your limited time. If you make your swim sessions count, however, you can achieve gains and still have sufficient time to commit to cycling and running.

#10 Embrace the base

The single most important phase of training is the base or Preparation Phase. This is the foundation upon which you build most of your aerobic and neuromuscular fitness.

The ultimate goal during this period is to execute consistent training in all three disciplines at a variety of intensities in order to hone general aerobic fitness. Consistency is absolutely essential in this Phase. It is only over the long term that your body adapts by conditioning muscles, building endurance and reducing the potential for injury once the load increases during the build or Specific Preparation/ Competition Phases of training.

From an efficiency perspective, the base is important because it prevents the need for cramming in exceptionally high-volume weeks. If you are continually engaged in steady base training, you are constantly honing your aerobic engine and are never far away from achieving a performance close to your maximum potential. Over the long term, consistency trumps erratic spikes in training volume and is less traumatic on the body.

You can actually race very well off of base fitness, assuming it is sufficiently broad. If you are a beginner, you should commit to approximately six months of base work before truly undertaking more aggressive training. If you are experienced, you can get by with less, assuming you do not take an exceptionally long break at the end of the season. One of the advantages of a well-structured and efficient training plan is that fatigue should never be exceptionally high at any one point and you should be able to resume base training shortly (approximately two weeks) after the final race of the season. This approach makes it easier for you to put in the kind of reliable training over the long term that will actually make you a better triathlete.

TLDR: Consistent, steady and well-structured base training over a period of months/years is one of, if not the, most important component of an effective and efficient training plan.

#11 Strive for appropriate body composition

In many cases, you can look at the field of competitors at the start of a race and predict who is going to be fast. This is because the greatest triathletes tend to look similar. They have relatively little body fat with muscles honed through miles of swimming, biking, running and a bit of weight training. Most are lean, but not necessarily lanky.

This is not a coincidence.

With the possible exception of the swim, carrying a lot of excess fat has a directly negative impact on performance. Assuming an athlete has sufficient muscle mass to generate power and enough fat to remain healthy, the strength of the most important physiological indicators that predict performance —including VO2 max, watts per kg, exercise economy, etc. — are inversely correlated with body mass. All things being equal, endurance racing is a test of how much power you can generate over a distance relative to your body weight. You can have the most elite respiratory and cardiovascular system in the world — your cardiac output and absolute maximal oxygen uptake could be extraordinary — but if you are carrying around a lot of extra fat, you are not going to be able to compete with the best. Put a 25-pound backpack on Jan Frodeno or Kenenisa Bekele and ask them to complete a race and suddenly you will see average Joes beating them — and that is assuming they do not get injured while their joints, bones and ligaments endure extra stress generated by the excessive pounding brought on by additional dead weight.

Although there is no perfect body composition, most elite male endurance athletes have a body fat percentage in the upper single digits, whereas females tend to be in the low to upper teens. They also tend to have a substantial amount of muscle — at least when compared to other endurance athletes like runners and cyclists — though this muscle is functional and there is little excess mass.

This is not to say that you cannot be heavy and finish races. If you post up at the finish of a large race, you will likely be amazed at the variety of athlete body types — old, chubby, short, tall, obese, thin — but if you want to be fast, you need to maximize your power to weight ratio. In fact, many triathletes would be better served dropping 10+ pounds than increasing training volume.

Think of it this way: for men, many people consider a functional threshold power — or number of watts one can hold for an hour on the bike — of four watts per kilogram to be a reasonable minimum target if an age grouper wishes to qualify for Kona. This is a rash overgeneralization, but it is often a benchmark or goal of aspiring qualifiers. A 200-pound (91 kg) person would need to be able to put out 364 watts for an hour to achieve an FTP of four watts per kilogram — a very high number and difficult without exceptional genetics. A 160-pound person (72 kg), however, only needs to put out 288 watts for an hour to achieve an FTP of 4 watts per kg — an impressive number certainly, but one that is much more realistic for average young or middle aged men to achieve. This is why it is rare (but not unheard of) for people carrying above ~2.4 lbs per inch (or 1.1 kg per inch) to reach elite levels in triathlon. Most elites are in the 2.0-2.40 lbs per inch range.

A few examples:

-**Daniela Ryf:** 5' 9", 139 lbs: 2.01 lbs per inch

-**Sarah True:** 5' 8", 137 lbs: 2.01 lbs per inch

-**Craig Alexander**: 5'11", 150 lbs: 2.11 lbs per inch

-**Lionel Sanders:** 5'10", 165 lbs: 2.36 lbs per inch

Even though top triathletes are leaner than the general population, it is important to remember that there is a fine line between appropriate body composition and being too thin. Even more detrimental than carrying a few extra pounds of fat and muscle is being malnourished. Triathlon is a sport where you need to generate power. If you do not have the strength to pull yourself through the water, put out watts on the bike or muscle through the final miles of the run with fatigued legs, you will not do well. When you become underweight, you lose the ability to recover from workouts and are more susceptible to illness and overtraining. If you are going to err, you should err on the side of being a bit heavier and STRONG than too light.

TLDR: If you want to be fast and stave off injury, you should strive for an appropriate weight/body composition for your gender. But do NOT strive to be underweight. Your performance will suffer.

Disclaimer: Body image issues and eating disorders are an enormous problem in endurance sports and one needs to be careful not to develop an unhealthy approach to eating and nutrition. A well-balanced diet is best. If you are looking for a cohesive nutrition plan, seek the counsel of a professional nutritionist.

Part 2
The Disciplines

Chapter 6

The Swim

How to structure swim training for maximum benefit

The swim portion of a triathlon is one which age group triathletes either love or hate. People who swam as children tend to wield an enormous advantage over adult onset swimmers, coming out of the water minutes ahead with seemingly little effort. Meanwhile, otherwise fit people (i.e., those with running or cycling backgrounds but no swim background) flail about, putting out tremendous energy while making very little forward progress. It is a remarkable phenomenon, the reason(s) for which triathletes have pondered for decades. Is it lack of work in the pool? Can one not learn how to swim correctly after a certain age?

The true answer lies somewhere in the middle, but the general ineptitude of many age group triathletes in the water continues to be the brunt of jokes from pure swimmers. If you swam as a child and participate in triathlons, you probably relish this ineptitude. Otherwise, you are probably looking to achieve a level of competency in the water that simply minimizes damage; though, hopefully, you are aiming a bit higher than mediocrity.

In this chapter, I'll explore the specific nature of the triathlon swim — analyzing its relative importance and the specific difficulties facing new or adult onset swimmers, the unique challenges they face and what they are doing wrong. I'll also look into what makes a good swimmer and how each type of swimmer – the experienced or novice – should approach swim training if they want to race faster with appropriate time investment. We'll also cover the best way for Maximus, Kim, Bill and Imogene to approach swim training.

How important is the swim?

The swim is a small, albeit important, component of triathlon. In long course, it might take up 10% of total time, whereas in an Olympic distance race it typically composes closer to 20%. Based on pure percentages, the swim has less of an impact on overall race time than the bike or run. This is not to say that the swim is not important, but if your goal is to become brutally efficient with training, you need to keep in mind that there is only so much time to be gained in the water and you need to make your training sessions count. If you do not put in your dues, you will lose many minutes to the athletes who spend time in the pool.

There is an often repeated quotation that says: "You can't win a triathlon with a swim, but you can certainly lose it." On the surface, the statement is obviously true. You cannot win a triathlon with a good swim because you still have to bike and run after. Duh. And you can certainly lose a triathlon due to a poor swim assuming your bike and run are not strong enough to make up the time you lose. But if we dig a bit deeper, we might actually find some wisdom in the quotation, specifically as it relates to how triathletes train for the swim and how so few devote the appropriate amount of time to it.

Finding the correct balance

Just as people either love or hate the swim, they often approach swim training in two polarized manners: they either commit way too much time and energy to it or not nearly enough. I know many triathletes who strive to swim five or six times a week. These are usually people who have swim backgrounds — perhaps they swam in high school or college — and they are used to the routine and incredible volume that top-level swimmers put in. This is fine if they enjoy it or have comparable free time to bike and run like many professionals; but, many of these people aspire to perform well in triathlons, must contend with busy schedules and do not realize just how little swim speed they would lose if they, for example, slashed their six 90-minute sessions to three high-quality 60-minute sessions and used the extra time to work on the bike and run. Their drop in swim performance would be infinitesimal.

61

Swim fitness and technique tends to linger much better and longer than bike or run fitness.

On the other side of the spectrum, we have the adult onset swimmers who, even after months of training, barely improve. These athletes usually have bike or run backgrounds and view the swim as a necessary evil and, as such, approach training with that mentality. They might only swim occasionally and, when they do, they simply slog through laps without focus. They do not embed enough deliberate swim work into their training plans to become competent in the water.

For both these groups, it is important to frame the importance of the swim and one's relative talents properly. For the great swimmer who already has the tools to do well, it makes sense to focus on maintenance and devote more time to the bike and run. Poor or adult onset swimmers, on the other hand, need to approach training with specific, laser-like focus to achieve a base level of competency, though this does not necessarily require an inordinate time investment either, assuming the approach attacks the unique challenges facing learning swimmers.

The phenomenon of the adult onset swimmer

Because of the pervasiveness of poor swimmers in triathlon, with the majority of these being adult onset swimmers, it is important to address the specific problems these athletes face. Far too often, triathletes approach swim training with little or no direction. They struggle in the water and after a period of time with little or minimal progress, they chock up their poor performance to having "low body fat" or "long runner legs." (Excuses which are complete rubbish) Nearly everyone can become a good swimmer if they approach training correctly and attack their problem areas. To do this requires doing what good swimmers do: paying unrelenting attention to technique, harnessing feedback from others, spending sufficient time in the water and structuring sessions appropriately. So before and after each swim session, ask yourself:

WHAT DO GOOD SWIMMERS DO?

#1 They focus on great technique

If you watch Olympic swimmers or top-level triathletes swim, you will see some variety in stroke technique. Some have straight arm recoveries and high turnover, while others have longer, slower, more powerful strokes. Certain variation is acceptable; however, there are two traits that most great swim strokes have and which you should place highest priority on developing: good body position and a propulsive catch. These two variables form the foundation of the stroke.

Good body position

All fast swimmers swim with their bodies parallel to the bottom of the pool. Their legs and feet are up near the surface as their head, shoulders, torso, waist and legs follow in suit through the water in a straight line, minimizing drag and frontal surface area. Their toes are pointed and their kick is compact, whether it is a two-beat or six-beat kick.

Common errors: The most common problem for poor swimmers is dragging legs and feet. You can remedy this by learning to float horizontally in the water. Practice by looking down at the bottom of the pool and tightening the glutes and hamstrings to lift your legs. Your core should be taut and your body should be elongated in a straight line. Focus on "pressing the buoy," which means you should visualize that the central point of flotation is actually your chest and you should consciously "press" your chest (or buoy) into the water in order to elevate your legs.

Perhaps the most common stroke flaw that leads to sinking legs is when swimmers raise their heads or lift their chins. When you lift your chin, either by looking ahead or breathing incorrectly, a see-saw effect occurs and your legs sink. To remedy this, keep your head in a neutral position, with your neck in alignment with your spine. When you breathe, try to keep one goggle in the water.

Drills: To fix sinking legs, emphasize side kicking with one goggle in the water, the superman drill, floating and kick and switch. Swimming with a snorkel is great for learning to keep your head down and developing good alignment. No matter what you're doing, always focus on keeping your head neutral—i.e. looking down at the bottom of the pool or slightly ahead.

A great catch

Apart from body position, the other important component of a good swim stroke is the catch. All fast swimmers have a good feel for the water and usually utilize an early vertical forearm (EVF). This means that when their lead hand enters the water and the arm is extended in front, their elbow remains fairly close to the surface while the hand and forearm drop to create a "paddle." The hand and forearm remain perpendicular to the surface as they "catch" or "grip" as much water as early in the stroke as possible so as to maximize the volume of water they purchase and throw behind them. By doing this, you can move more forcefully and efficiently through the water.

Common errors: Many poor swimmers drop their elbow, causing their arm and hand to slip through the water. If you find your hand slipping, you should focus intently on developing an early vertical forearm and "grabbing" as much water as possible early in every stroke cycle. Try to maintain a sensation of pressure on your hand and forearm as you push water directly backwards towards your feet.

Drills: Single Arm Freestyle is probably the best drill for developing a good catch. Other great drills include fist, catch up, pulling with paddles, and sculling to develop feel for the water.

Other stroke variables

Achieving good body position and strengthening your catch may seem like simple concepts, but they can be very difficult to achieve. Although there are certainly other important areas to devote focus, such as hand entry, kick technique, stroke rate, etc., if you obsessively focus on perfecting body position and catch first, you will become a better swimmer sooner than if you attempted to work on every little detail simultaneously. The best swimmers have developed these two areas with hours upon hours of focused and deliberate practice. It may feel awkward or difficult at the beginning, but by mentally engaging around maintaining a streamlined body position and working on achieving an EVF and strong catch, you will develop specific strength and motor skills so that an effective and faster stroke becomes second nature. Once this happens, it will be easier to make other stroke adjustments, leading to further marginal gains.

Swim Drills

Above all, spending time in the water and being engaged with your stroke will allow you to get faster. Swim drills, if you know how to do them correctly, can be useful for developing a feel for the water and improving technique, but don't fall into the trap of thinking that doing drills for 80% of the duration of your swim sessions will magically make you faster. To progress, you need to swim a lot and focus on nailing the fundamentals. However, drills like single arm freestyle, catch up, fist, kicking, swimming with a snorkel, pulling, fingertip drag, kick and switch and sculling can be great for remaining engaged and developing a feel for the water. Pick a couple each session and do them as part of your pre-set. To learn how to do these drills, head over to www.workingtriathlete.com/resources and click the swim drills link.

#2 They seek feedback from others

Swimming well requires tremendous body awareness and feel for the water. Unfortunately, especially for newer swimmers, this innate feel is lacking and it can be difficult to know what one looks like while swimming and what corrections are needed. It may feel like you are rhythmically swimming through the water like a dolphin when in reality you are splashing about inefficiently. If you are doing something wrong and do not correct it, you will engrain that poor technique into your muscle memory, making it more difficult to correct later on. This is why it is important to get feedback from knowledgeable individuals such as swim instructors/coaches who know what a good stroke looks like and who can make recommendations to fix form flaws.

One readily accessible avenue via which to receive swim instruction is through your local Masters Swim group. Most cities have locations that offer Masters Practices for all ability levels that are led by experienced coaches who are more than willing to critique your stroke technique. You will also have other swimmers there to push you as you execute structured practices and learn the more nuanced aspects of swim training (drills, various strokes, flip turns, etc.). Getting feedback from coaches and other swimmers will allow you to progress at a much faster rate than if you tried to do it all yourself. When you are looking to make your sessions count, I highly recommend you do it with a Masters Swim group. You simply cannot do it as efficiently on your own.

#3 They spend time in the water

Even if you know exactly what a good stroke looks like and have decent body awareness, you will never build endurance and achieve a fast swim time if you do not actually swim. The combination of technique development and time in the water is what will make you faster. The stroke is not natural and the muscles required to swim fast are not normally used in everyday life, so it is important to stimulate them and develop the coordination, fitness and neural connections that will allow you to maintain good technique even when you are tired.

Although the fast swimmers that so many triathletes envy likely had years of 90-minute, two-a-day swim sessions, this volume is neither sustainable nor practical for a working three-sport athlete. Instead, you should focus on frequency and density within sessions. Aim for at least three workouts per week if you are a relatively poor swimmer. Four is better. These sessions do not have to be long (30-45 minutes is fine depending on your goals and availability), but you need to be consistent and hyper-focused while in the water. You should be mentally engaged with every stroke, focusing on body position and a good catch.

#4 They know their threshold pace and structure their workouts appropriately

Swim training is markedly different from cycling and running in that swimmers rarely perform long continuous swims. Because swimming is a relatively low-impact exercise and form is so important, the underlying wisdom is that, even for individuals training for longer distances, swim workouts composed almost exclusively of intervals with frequent rest is desirable. This allows you to swim at relatively high intensity for a larger chunk of the workout and, perhaps more importantly, the frequent short rests allow you to recover a bit, thereby preventing your technique from breaking down.

Even for long course racing, doing work around or faster than your threshold pace on a consistent basis is essential for maximizing swim performance. As I described in the Nitty Gritty chapter, there are many ways to determine your threshold pace; the most straightforward of which is swimming an all-out 1000 yard/meter time trial. Your pace per 100 yards/meters is your threshold pace. Another option for less experienced swimmers is swimming 3X300 yards/meters with 30 seconds rest between each. The average pace of the intervals is your threshold pace.

Following is an explanation of swim intensity zones:

Swim Training Zones

Zone 1

RPE: 1 to 2

Purpose: Active Recovery

Swim pace per 100: Easy or technique

Zone 2

RPE: 3-4 **Purpose:** Endurance

Swim pace per 100: T-Pace plus 10 seconds

Zone 3

RPE: 5-6 **Purpose:** Tempo

Swim pace per 100: T-Pace plus 5 seconds

Zone 4

RPE: 7-8 **Purpose:** Threshold

Swim pace per 100: T-Pace

Zone 5

RPE: 9-10 **Purpose:** VO2 Max

Swim pace per 100: T-Pace minus 5 seconds

How to establish and utilize swim zones

Assume you swam the 1000 yard time trial in 20 minutes. This means that your threshold or T pace is 2:00 per 100 yards. So if you were looking to do Zone 5 intervals, you would aim to maintain a pace of 1:55 (2:00 − 5 seconds = 1:55).

Swim sessions

Swim practices are notorious for being complicated. The jargon and abbreviations used to describe swim workouts can become laughably difficult for a beginner swimmer. In reality, effective swim sessions do not need to take up a whole white board to describe (though variety can be nice to break up the monotony!). For sake of simplicity, most swim workouts can be effectively structured as follows:

-**Warm-up** (can be short—five minutes of easy swimming)

-**Pre-set with drills** (optional if time-strapped — can be as simple as 3X100 alternating drills every 50)

-**Main-set** (straightforward intervals totaling 1,000-2,000+ yards)

-**Cool-down** (optional if time strapped — I usually prescribe an easy 100-400 pull).

The main-set is really the only non-negotiable component of the workout. Other components are beneficial but can be abbreviated or eliminated if you do not have time. Ideally, you would do a brief warm-up and a pre-set with drills (if you know how to do them correctly and they have a purpose) along with a main-set and cool-down. If you are on your own, simpler is better. Incredibly complicated sessions are not more effective than something like 15x100 on 15 seconds rest or 30x50 on the minute. Working on strokes that are not freestyle can be useful for developing feel for the water, but if you are short on time, simply focus on freestyle. You will use it exclusively in races.

If you remain focused, you can knock out an effective session in 30-60 minutes quite easily. If you perform three of these sessions each week, your total time commitment could be less than two or three hours — resulting in volume much less than that of most pure swimmers, but more than enough to make you proficient in the water. After you develop a foundation, you can maintain competency with as little as two workouts a week, although I typically recommend that true beginners or adult onset swimmers aim for at least three or four sessions a week in order to more effectively hardwire neurons to execute the stroke correctly. Due to the diminishing return on time investment, very good swimmers would likely be better served shooting for two or three sessions a week.

Types of Sessions (main-sets)

Because your overall volume will be fairly low, there will be no such thing as recovery swims. Every swim should include a bit of intensity, even if it is just 4x25 at the end of the workout. I like to split most workouts into either endurance or muscular endurance classifications, with the occasional open water race simulation. You should aim to do at least one of each every week.

Endurance Sets

Endurance sets are predominately in Zones 2-3 and are composed of longer intervals of 200-500 meter/yards with short rest. The goal of these workouts is to maximize volume with good technique.

Example endurance sets:

-3X400, 4X200 building from Zone 2 to Zone 3 with 30 seconds rest. Distance per stroke for 200s.

-500, 400, 300, 200, 100 Zone 2 building to Zone 4 with 20 seconds rest.

Muscular Endurance Sets

Muscular endurance sets emphasize higher-intensity swimming in Zones 4-5 and are comprised of shorter intervals of 25-200 meters/yards. These workouts are intended to build strength, power and promote good form at a high effort.

Example muscular endurance sets:

-20x50 Zone 5 with 20 seconds rest

-6x150 Zone 4 with 30 seconds rest

Open Water/Race Simulation

Because most triathlons have open water swims, it is absolutely essential to get comfortable swimming in natural bodies of water. Swimming in lakes, rivers, bays and the ocean is entirely different than swimming in chlorinated pools. In open water races, there is chop, it is dark, there are no walls and there are often dozens of other athletes thrashing about around you. You need to prepare for these variables. I often encourage athletes to swim with others during open water practice swims not only for safety, but also to practice drafting and getting comfortable swimming in close quarters with others. These workouts are also a good time to focus on tactics (sighting, drafting, turning at buoys, etc.) and emphasizing longer sets, sometimes even the full race distance.

Time Hacks

-Do not obsess over the warm-up or cool-down. Ensure you are warm by swimming a couple of easy laps, but do not turn it into a 15-minute leisurely floating session. Cool-downs, when time-strapped, can be skipped.

-Remain focused on nailing the main-set. Do not dawdle between intervals. Keep the rest short.

-Make your sessions count by swimming with a Masters Swim group.

-Do not underestimate the productivity of a 30-minute, focused swim session.

-One of the most economical ways to execute training is via swim-bricks, especially a swim/run or swim/strength session. For example, assuming your pool is at a typical workout facility, you can do a 30-minute swim and 30-minute strength or run session in an hour all under one roof.

-Focus on swimming. Toys like fins and kick boards have their place and should be integrated intelligently, but if you are looking to be brutally efficient and gain swim fitness, focus on the fundamentals.

How Maximus, Kim, Bill and Imogene successfully approached triathlon swim training

Maximus the magnificent swimmer

Maximus was already a strong swimmer when we started working with him. As a D1 swimmer in college, he was borderline Olympic trials caliber. So when he came to us with the goal of completing an iron distance as soon as feasible, it was clear that his lack of cycling/run experience and fitness were going to be the limiters and that a disproportionate amount of time should be committed to them. For many time-strapped athletes (especially proficient swimmers), it makes sense to cut the number of swim sessions back to as few as two per week. Maximus, however, wanted to retain as much of his swim ability as possible (not that it really would have gone anywhere), and it was clear that having an exceptionally fast swim would boost his confidence. For this reason, we only cut the number of swim sessions back to three per week, allowing him to unleash an incredible swim at his A-Race and earning a first out of the water award. All the sessions were targeted, high density workouts that lasted 60 minutes.

Kim the corporate executive

With her eyes set on completing a half iron distance race, it was essential for Kim to develop strength and endurance in the water. Since she could only workout once per day, we limited her swims to Monday, Wednesday and Friday and followed all of them with a run or strength training session. Her swims lingered around the 2,000 meter mark, which was sufficient distance to develop very good fitness for the 1.2 mile swim, but sufficiently short to allow for a subsequent session (she would be done in ~45 minutes).

Bill the older uber biker

For Bill, like with most adult onset swimmers, the swim was a challenge. Since at first he was unable to swim very far during each session, it was clear that he needed to swim frequently so as to accrue time in the water and progress. Because of this, we aimed for five, very short (30 minutes or less) swim sessions each week that included drills to develop comfort and feel for the water. All intervals for the first month were 100 yards or less (usually less). By being hyper-focused on form and joining a Masters swim group, Bill was able to progress rapidly (all things considered) and was able to swim a mile non-stop within two months. For his first sprint triathlon, the swim was the least of his worries.

Imogene the artist

Imogene had a very solid stroke when we started to work with her. Her comfort in the water was strong from the beginning and, as such, she had an advantage over adult onset swimmers like Bill. For Imogene, the goal was to simply execute a balanced swim regimen and work on building strength and endurance in the water via a key intensity, key endurance, and form/hybrid session each week. By swimming three times per week, she was able to swim in the top 10-percent of her age group at her first tri and was not phased by having to swim in the ocean during her first off-road triathlon.

The bottom line: view the swim as part of a larger training strategy

As you may have realized, appropriate training is not a one-size fits all endeavor. You need to be honest with your strengths and weaknesses and realistic about your relative potential for improvement within various areas. Depending on your situation, you may be better served by swimming more than the bare minimum. Triathlon training is about strategically balancing time investment in areas that will lead to the greatest times savings on race day.

Chapter 7

The Bike

It's not all about the bike—but it mostly is

The importance of the cycling leg in triathlon

For most triathletes, the bike portion of training is the most time consuming — and for good reason. It is, arguably, the most important component. In almost every triathlon distance, the bike encompasses the largest portion of the race. In long course racing, it typically accounts for over 50% of race time and in sprints/Olympics, it comprises slightly under that. There is, quite simply, a lot of time to be gained or lost on the bike.

But bike fitness is not just important for laying down a good cycling time; it also has a direct impact on your run. Having the ability to come off the bike fairly fresh is essential for running well. Poor cyclists tend to have triathlon run times far slower than their open race times, whereas stellar cyclists can lay down run times fairly close to their open race times. It does not matter if you are the best runner in the world: if you come off the bike and your legs feel like Jell-o, you are not going to run well.

For Bill, emphasizing the bike allowed him to execute high intensity training while avoiding injury. For Kim and Maximus, it allowed them to persevere through 56 and 112 miles respectively and feel good at the start of the run. For Imogene, increasing cycling strength allowed her to ride on technical mountain biking trails and enjoy cycling more.

Because of its importance and benefits, it is imperative to train properly for the bike and to understand what the cycling leg of triathlon requires.

The nature of the cycling leg

In most triathlons, the bike portion is essentially an individual time trial, meaning you are not allowed to draft. There are draft-legal races (ITU races being the most popular), but the vast majority of triathlons are non-draft races where you must maintain a certain distance behind other riders so as not to benefit from their slipstream, which can save up to 30-40% in energy expenditure. Depending on the organizing body overseeing the race, the gap you have to maintain varies, typically in the realm of three to six bike lengths. The ramifications of this are that you do not really have to be concerned with various strategies that pervade draft-legal races — such as sprinting, covering breakaways, etc. It is a wholly individual endeavor. As such, most triathletes should approach cycling training with the intention of building an engine that allows for the highest steady power output appropriate for a given distance. In nearly every case, this will lead to the fastest time relative to effort expended.

What not to do: how many people approach cycling training

Many people take the "longer is better" approach to cycling, meaning that more saddle time leads to better performance. They strive to execute multiple long easy rides each week with the sole focus of maximizing the number of hours they enter into their training logs. They view their long weekend group ride as an indispensable staple of training. They think a ride of less than an hour is useless and, as such, they ride infrequently (<3 time per week) due to time constraints. Unless they are actually ascending a hill, many athletes never ride hard.

This is not an appropriate approach for a busy triathlete who wishes to race fast.

For pure cyclists, frequent long easy rides have their place, but this is because they have the luxury of committing all their training hours to solely cycling and these easy rides are in addition to the "meat" of training, which is a steady diet of intervals, hills and threshold riding. Sure, logging hundreds of miles of leisurely riding does lead to positive aerobic adaptations—relentless volume, if you can handle it, can make up for a lot of training errors; however, when you have two other sports to train for — sports that already add to overall aerobic volume — you need to focus on that which will make you faster on race day. This means emphasizing workouts that efficiently raise your fitness: i.e., high-benefit, low-cost sessions.

What to do: how you should approach cycling training

Fortunately or unfortunately, depending on your perspective or love for pain, the nature of cycling allows you to push yourself on a consistent basis with relatively little recovery cost. Cycling is unique in that it is low-impact, meaning it is not particularly traumatic on your connective tissues. Assuming your bike fits you well, there is a low risk of injury due to overuse. You can certainly ramp up your saddle time or intensity too quickly but, relative to running, you should be able to sustain a higher volume/intensity without hurting yourself or burning out. As the "you need to stop pedaling easy" principle implies, working triathletes looking to gain cycling fitness as efficiently as possible should spend much of their time at higher intensities by doing shorter, more frequent workouts.

How to do it: understanding cycling metrics and intensities

To boost cycling fitness, you need to understand the purpose of training and develop a plan that includes specific workouts at appropriate times within the training cycle. To achieve this, you need a metric to key off of so that you execute workouts at appropriate intensities — the most important of which is your functional threshold power, or FTP.

As we covered in the Nitty Gritty chapter, FTP is the highest average power (in watts) that you can maintain for an hour. The reason FTP is important is because it is used to determine your training zones, workout intensities and target race power. Most training plans prescribe workouts relative to your FTP. For example, if your FTP is 200 watts, a workout might prescribe 2X20 minutes at 95% of your FTP, or

190 watts. If you are conservatively racing a 70.3, you might want to target 75% of your FTP, or 150 watts. In this manner, once you know your FTP, you know exactly what power to hit for each interval and can execute workouts and races with precision.

Fortunately, it is easy to determine your FTP and you do not actually have to go all out for an hour each time you test in order to get a reasonably accurate assessment. As described earlier, the easiest way to establish your FTP is to warm up for approximately 20-30 minutes and perform a five minute interval close to all out. After a short recovery, ride as hard as you can for 20 minutes, tracking your average power over this 20 minute effort. Take that average power and subtract 5%. This is your FTP.

To establish your heart rate at threshold power, measure your average heart rate over an interval during which you aim to maintain 100% of your FTP. The point at which your heart rate stabilizes is your threshold heart rate (THR). You can also determine your threshold heart rate by tracking your average heart rate during a 45 to 60-minute race effort, or by doing a solo, 30-minute all-out time trial. Your average heart rate over the last 20 minutes of the effort is your THR.

By establishing your THR, you can deduce what your heart rate within various zones should be and you can determine how your heart rate correlates to your power output within various zones. Additionally, if you do not have a power meter (either because you choose not to ride with one or it breaks during a ride/race), you can use THR to get an approximate estimate of your effort independent of rated perceived exertion.

Following is a list of zones along with the training purpose and associated power and heart rate targets within each. The metrics are specific to cycling, but are similar in concept to those used in running.

Cycling Training Zones

Zone 1

RPE: 1 to 2 **Purpose:** Active Recovery

Bike % FTP: <55% **Bike % THR:** <69%

Zone 2

RPE: 3-4 **Purpose:** Endurance

Bike % FTP: 56-75% **Bike % THR**: 69-83%

Zone 3

RPE: 5-6 **Purpose:** Tempo

Bike % FTP: 76-90% **Bike % THR**: 84-94%

Zone 4

RPE: 7-8 **Purpose:** Threshold

Bike % FTP: 91-105% **Bike % THR**: 95-105%

Zone 5

RPE: 9-10 **Purpose:** VO2 Max

Bike % FTP: 106-120% **Bike % THR**: >105%

How to use these metrics

In following up on our earlier example, assume you averaged 200 watts for your 20 minute FTP test. This means that your FTP is 190. To determine your Zone 3 target power range, multiply 190 by 76% and 90% (190 X .76 = 144; 190 X .90 = 171) to get a target wattage range of 144-171 watts.

To determine your target heart rate within various zones, follow the same protocol. For example, if you established your threshold heart rate to be 150 BPM and are looking to determine your Zone 2 target heart rate range, multiply 150 by 69% and 83% to get a range of 104-125 BPM.

Recognize that your heart rate can vary day to day and is impacted by fatigue, temperature and other factors. Everyone's relative heart rate is different and your average heart rate within each zone can actually vary between disciplines. For example, people with a strong running background may have a higher heart rate while running in Zone 5 versus when they cycle in Zone 5. Also note that your heart has a delayed response to various efforts, which is why measuring power is usually a superior and more objective method for measuring exertion in real-time.

Breaking down the zones

Apart from knowing your cycling intensity zones, you should understand their respective purposes, the benefits within each and which ones to target most often.

Zone 1—Active Recovery

This is easy riding. You should be able to easily talk or even sing while in this zone and your heart rate and power should be low. Its purpose is to simply stimulate blood flow. Apart from warming up, cooling down or flushing out lactate, a working triathlete striving for efficiency will not spend a whole lot of time at this intensity. A lot of easy group rides default to this effort.

Zone 2—Endurance

This is an important zone and the majority of your overall easy base/supporting mileage should be at this effort. You should be able to speak in full sentences and maintain the pace for hours. Its purpose is to build your aerobic engine by improving, among other things, fat utilization, lactate clearance and mitochondrial density. Athletes, especially beginners, need to spend a lot of time in this zone before integrating harder workouts as it is vital for developing the aerobic foundation upon which fitness is built.

Zone 3—Tempo

This zone often gets a bad rap from those who advocate polarized training since they argue that time in Zone 3 does not deliver substantial benefit in excess of Zone

2, nor does it deliver benefit equal to Zone 4. It is essentially the "middle child" of intensity zones. This claim is debatable and is really more applicable to running where recovery costs are higher and pounding the pavement in Zone 3 each day would compromise recovery and inhibit execution of key workouts. Considering the lower recovery cost of cycling, however, and the fact that many races require mostly Zone 3 efforts, it does hold an important place in a well-structured training plan. In fact, a definitive exception to the "avoid Zone 3" rule is the undeniable benefits of upper Zone 3 (~85-93% of FTP), which is part of the "sweetspot zone" and can deliver adaptations and advantages similar to Zone 4 with lower recovery costs.

Zone 4—Threshold

One of the most important zones for building cycling fitness, Zone 4 is around your threshold power — or the power you can maintain for an hour. It is a hard effort that many inexperienced riders underestimate. In theory, your FTP is directly below the point at which your body produces more lactate than it can clear. Workouts performed in and around this zone do a great job of raising your FTP and, by association, your overall cycling fitness.

Zone 5—VO2 Max/Aerobic Capacity

Exhausting but incredibly effective for gaining and sharpening high-end fitness, Zone 5 is near your VO2 max, or the highest power/pace at which your body can function aerobically. You should only be in this zone during hard intervals — typically intervals of one to five minutes separated by recovery periods. These efforts are very challenging and are reflective of your body's ability to deliver oxygen to working muscles. Thus, Zone 5 efforts are dependent on the strength of your heart (e.g., stroke volume), capillary density, hemoglobin and muscle cell composition (e.g., mitochondrion size, aerobic enzymes, etc.). Time in this zone efficiently improves these adaptations, though recovery costs can be high.

Zone 6—Anaerobic Capacity

The most intense efforts, or those classified as anaerobic efforts, fall into Zone 6. This zone is useful for neuromuscular work or maximizing muscle recruitment for sprinters. Although fine on occasion, there is little need for most triathletes to spend much time in this zone.

Putting it all together: what to focus on

When structuring an effective, time-efficient plan, it is important to keep the larger picture in mind. As I mentioned, your goal as a triathlete, especially in the Preparation Phase, should be to increase your FTP. This is important because it is easily measurable, reflects your ability to lay down high and steady watts —which is precisely what triathlons require you to do — and directly relates to your aerobic zones; in other words, if you increase your FTP, your Zone 1, 2, 3 and 5 power and pace will also increase.

I should clarify that FTP is not everything, though the correlation between a higher one and a faster bike split is VERY strong. There are other indicators, such as the duration for which one can hold Z3 tempo or sweetspot efforts comfortably, which may serve as superior metrics for establishing preparedness for certain races such as half irons; however, FTP is such a universal and readily measureable heuristic to gauge cycling fitness that it makes sense to emphasize it. To claim otherwise is to be pedantic for abstruse reasons. FTP matters. A lot.

The core cycling workouts

The most economical way to boost your functional threshold power is with frequent high-intensity sessions. You should shoot for at least three to four cycling workouts per week and most of these should last under an hour with an emphasis on sweetspot and threshold efforts. Following are examples of various workouts that form the core of an effective and time-efficient training plan.

Sweetspot Training (SST)

For time-strapped athletes, sweetspot (SST) workouts are the most essential for boosting cycling fitness. They should be your bread and butter. Since overall volume is sufficiently low in plans tailored to working triathletes, I often prescribe sweetspot rides in place of typical "supporting" or "steady" rides that other plans might prescribe. These should be executed early and often throughout the entire macrocycle. These workouts contain intervals in upper Zone 3, which is approximately 85-93% of your FTP. Spending time in this zone is markedly less taxing on the body than spending it at FTP, so recovery costs are lower but the benefit is still high. The effort should feel comfortably hard—around the max pace you could maintain for two hours; so certainly not easy, but not acutely grueling either. There are many ways to structure a sweetspot workout, though the most common way is via moderately long (10-40 minute) intervals, or by combining SST with short, higher-intensity bursts. Depending on your fitness level, it is not unreasonable to spend one to two hours at sweetspot intensity (typically broken up) and still recover fairly quickly, though most sessions will include 30-60 minutes of targeted work.

-Example SST Workout: Warm up 10 minutes starting in Zone 1 and ramping up to Zone 3; ride at 85-93% of your FTP for 40 minutes; 10-minute Zone 2 cool-down. Alternatively, replace the 40 minute effort with two 25-minute efforts separated by a short (1-5 minute) recovery interval.

Variations: Warm up 10 minutes starting in Zone 1 and ramping up to Zone 3; alternate 2 minutes at 85% of FTP and 10 seconds at 125% FTP for 25-30 minutes total; 5-10-minute Zone 2 cool-down.

FTP Intervals

FTP Intervals are similar in structure to sweetspot sessions, though they are executed in Zone 4. They are extremely effective at raising your FTP and have a lower cost than high-intensity VO2 workouts. These should be done weekly and are composed of intervals at or very close to your FTP — typically 95-100% of FTP. The most notorious workout is 2x20 minutes, which is simply two 20-minute intervals at around your FTP separated by a short recovery period (3-5 min) sandwiched between a warm-up and cool-down. Variations include 3x15 minutes or over-under workouts wherein you spend a few minutes of each interval riding 5-20 watts above and below your FTP. Depending on your fitness level and position within the macrocycle, you want to spend a total of 30-60 minutes in Z4 when you execute these sessions. Some examples:

   - Beginner/Quick FTP workout: Warm up 10 minutes starting in Zone 1 and ramping up to Zone 3; 15 minutes at 95% of your FTP; 5 minute recovery spin; 15 minutes at 95% of your FTP; 5-10 minute Zone 2 cool-down.

   -Advanced: Add an additional 15 minute interval to the Beginner/Quick FTP workout or increase the duration of the intervals to 20-30 minutes.

   -Variations: Feel free to get creative. Consider 4x10 minute intervals at 102% of your FTP with short (2 to 3 minute) rest or breaking your intervals into minute chunks wherein one minute is spent at 102-105% of your FTP followed by two minutes at 90-95% of your FTP, alternating throughout the duration of the interval.

VO₂ Intervals

Some of the more arduous sessions on the bike will be VO2 intervals. These are workouts where you execute repetitions in Zone 5, or at 105-120% of your FTP. The duration of the intervals should be fairly short — two to eight minutes depending on intensity. These should be fierce, with the first part of each interval feeling fairly hard, the middle part feeling difficult, and the latter part feeling close to all out.

VO2 intervals are essential for boosting your VO2 max: the maximum amount of oxygen your body can process. The higher your VO2 max, the higher you can raise your FTP, since FTP is limited by your ability to utilize oxygen at high workloads. Although these sessions are high-cost, they are also high-benefit and should be incorporated on a fairly consistent basis —every 7-10 days in some form throughout a macrocycle and more often when executing block training or in the build up to a sprint triathlon.

Beginner VO2 Workout: Warm up 10 minutes starting in Zone 1 and build to Zone 3; do 4x4 minute intervals with four minutes of recovery between each, with the first one being at 105% of your FTP and the others between 110% and 120%; 10-minute Zone 2 cool-down. As you get fitter, add additional intervals, vary the duration and shorten the rest periods. You typically should not spend over 30 minutes at VO2 effort throughout a workout, and 20 minutes or less is, in most cases, sufficient for generating a solid stimulus.

Key Endurance/Long Rides

Long rides are essential to a well-rounded training plan, but most people approach them incorrectly. Many view a long ride as a ride of well over four hours at an easy effort in Zone 1 or lower Zone 2. Although long easy rides of five to seven hours are beneficial in some respects, such as for testing sustainability of your bike position, honing in on a nutrition plan for long course racing and building aerobic fitness, you can achieve a similar physiological benefit by integrating higher intensity training closer to race pace into a "shorter" long ride of 2.5 to 4 hours.

You can structure a long ride in many different ways, including inserting two or three 20-minute sweetspot intervals in the middle or riding an hour or two at your 70.3 pace (~80% of your FTP) while attacking any hills. The rest of the ride should be in upper Zone 2.

Note that if you are training for long course triathlons, you will benefit from rides longer than three or four hours, if only for the psychological boost. I would recommend a couple of rides over 80 miles for your own confidence, but assuming you execute multiple "long" rides of approximately three hours that contain intervals at 80-95% FTP, you should feel relatively comfortable maintaining a typical iron distance power of 65-75% over the full 112 miles even if you did not execute a training ride of the same distance or duration.

Key Endurance Ride Example: 30 minutes in Zone 2; 2x20 minutes at 85% FTP with 10-minute recovery; remainder of ride at 75-80% FTP to equal 3 hours. Other example: 30 minute ramp to Z3; maintain 78-82% of your FTP for two additional hours.

Cycling within the macrocycle

Although everyone is different and a boiler-plate triathlon plan is not ideal for anyone, there are certain guidelines that you, as a time-strapped working triathlete, should follow as you move through a macrocycle. This includes emphasizing frequency and embracing appropriate high-benefit workouts, such as FTP and sweetspot sessions composed of long intervals (15-40 minutes) as well as other sessions that integrate a bit of VO2 work along with, when practical or necessary, longer endurance rides. In the General Preparation Subphase, the overall load should be less than in the Specific Preparation or Pre-Competition Subphases so as to avoid burnout and allow for recovery. However, because overall volume is never exceptionally high, you can and should continue to execute lower-volume, high-intensity workouts throughout the whole macrocycle.

Following is an explanation of what your cycling training should look like throughout a typical macrocycle.

Preparation Phase (usually 8-16+ weeks)

Although your level of experience is a large governor of the specifics of your cycling training in the Preparation Phase, the goal in the early part of the phase should be developing overall cycling fitness and strength. This is done with a short mesocycle of Zone 2-3 work that includes intervals of increasing intensity and duration and an emphasis on low-cadence work to develop muscular strength. As the General Preparation Subphase continues, your load continuously increases and you should integrate longer sweetspot and Zone 4 intervals as well as occasional VO2 intervals. For our highest load athletes, this can mean building up to either 30 minutes of VO2 work, 60 minutes at threshold, or two hours at sweetspot (all separated into intervals) in a single session. Most can race near their potential by building to 2/3 this volume.

In the Specific Preparation Subphase, you should continue with consistent Zone 3-5 work to nurture and grow general fitness while also incorporating workouts that focus on race simulation in a more targeted manner. This can include an emphasis on increasing the duration of your key endurance ride if you are training for a long course race or on boosting your higher intensity Zone 5 capabilities if you are training for a sprint triathlon.

Competition Phase (usually 6-10+ weeks)

In the Pre-Competition Subphase, you should continue emphasizing race-specific work. The overall load may plateau or decrease in anticipation of a series of races, but especially early on, assuming you have been adhering to the Working Triathlete training approach, you will not and should not need to substantially cut your training volume.

As the core Competition Subphase begins, you will need to focus on balancing racing and recovery with fitness maintenance. Training may become even more polarized in this phase. If you only have one or two key races for which you are training, you should maintain a comparable load throughout the Competition Phase up until you commence your taper — which should last approximately two weeks. The taper should entail an approximately 20% reduction in volume two weeks out from your goal race and another 20% in the final week. You should, however, still incorporate brief bouts of Zone 4 and 5 intensities throughout the taper so as not to lose touch with the neuromuscular demands of harder efforts.

Transition Phase (usually 2-4 weeks)

As described in prior chapters, after your final race you should engage in a couple of weeks of rest or active recovery. Do not perform any structured cycling workouts in this period. Feel free to enjoy some easy spins if you want, but keep the intensity very light.

A note on travel

When you travel, it can be difficult or impossible to bring your bike with you. If you have a sales or similar job that requires you to drive locally (i.e. not fly) and stay at hotels, you can simply bring your bicycle with you and set it up on a trainer in your hotel room or in the fitness center. Alternatively, you can use the spin bike in the fitness center or at the local gym. Although spin/stationary bikes utilize slightly different muscles than you use when cycling on your actual bike, the experience is more similar than different and you will reap comparable benefits. If, like Imogene, you're the kind of person who enjoys spin classes, do not be afraid to integrate them intelligently into the plan. Although not as efficient as pure cycling, they can be a good way to gain fitness if you like dancing on the bike and it's easy to find a studio in every large city.

An alternative approach that I use with many athletes is to concentrate key cycling sessions before and after a business trip and to focus on running while traveling. This might not be feasible if you travel four or more days in a row on a weekly basis, in which case you need to find a bike while you're away, but if most of your trips are short, stressing out about finding one in an unfamiliar city might not be worth the costs.

Racing

As previously mentioned, in most of your triathlon races, you will be riding solo without the benefit of drafting off of other riders. Although there are times you may have to race the field irrespective of the power you are generating, it is usually most efficient to maintain a steady power output during a race (note that if the course is rolling, there could be a benefit to applying slightly more power on the uphills and slightly less on the downhills, but be careful not to burn too many matches. A lower variability in power is usually the best approach). In this regard, you should harness data, such as heart rate and power, to ensure that you are riding at appropriate intensities. The following are general power guidelines that most fit individuals can follow during various race distances. It is important to remember that faster/fitter people can complete each distance at a higher percentage of their threshold power because they are racing for a shorter period of time, so if you are a beginner or slower rider, err on targeting the lower end of the recommendations. If you are well-trained and faster, consider pushing the upper limits:

-**Sprint Distance** (~20K): 90-105% or Zone 4 to 5

-**Olympic Distance** (~40K): 90-95% or upper Zone 3 to lower Zone 4

-**Half Iron Distance** (~56 miles): 75%-90% or Zone 3

-**Full Iron Distance** (~112 miles) 65%-80% or Zone 2 to lower Zone 3

In training, you should be aware of the effort you are exerting and how it relates to your ideal race pace. This will allow you to determine your rate of perceived exertion at various intensities, which will enable you to race intuitively without needing to constantly check your power meter. You should also be aware of unique race conditions and how they might impact your ability to hold your theoretical ideal wattage. This is especially true in hot races where you may need to adjust your target power down 5-10% or more to prevent your body and brain from shutting down. Always harness all data available to you: power, heart rate and RPE to ensure that you are maximizing your race performance relative to the conditions and your physiological status on any given day.

How Maximus, Kim, Bill and Imogene successfully approached cycling training

Maximus the magnificent swimmer

Maximus took quite well to the bike, enjoying a fairly high FTP immediately. As someone who could recover quite well from intense sessions, we were able to integrate frequent Z4 and Z5 sessions that he usually completed late at night on the trainer in his New York apartment. He did 95% of his rides on the trainer, including some 4+hour rides in preparation for his first iron distance race. This approach enabled him to lay down a sub-5 hour bike split and feel good enough to run a stellar marathon.

Typically, Maximus completed four cycling workouts a week, including one key intensity session (Z4-5), one moderate intensity session (SST, Z3-4), one steady aerobic ride when time allowed (Upper Z2) and a longer ride with intervals (2+hours) on the weekends. During the initial months, as with most athletes, we focused on boosting FTP and aerobic capacity and as his key iron distance race approached, made sure he had the endurance and tactical savviness to execute on race day.

Kim the corporate executive

For Kim, efficiency was paramount. Like Maximus, she did most of her sessions on the indoor trainer. She typically rode three times per week, on Tuesday, Thursday and Sunday. Tuesday was the key intensity session and was often composed of Z4 intervals followed by a short run. Thursday was another fairly intense session that usually contained sweetspot or tempo efforts and Sunday was her long ride.

Although we strove to maximize cycling volume, Kim's overall cycling load was a bit lower than we might typically target for athletes with her level of motivation, talent and durability, simply because we had to adhere to the morning brick structure so that her evenings were free. Most of her rides were immediately followed or preceded by a run, so we had to consider the aggregate physical impact of these sessions and adjust down the load to account for this structure. Nevertheless, the approach was the same: a steady diet of targeted workouts with a lot of the riding spent in Z3/4 in order to efficiently develop fitness and, subsequently, a persistent focus on race-specific (half iron intensity) cycling efforts and tactics.

Bill the older uber biker

As an older gentleman with a strong cycling background, we immediately allocated almost all of Bill's weekly intensity to the bike (his run load was almost all Z2 in order to stave off injury). Since there is evidence that aerobic capacity diminishes disproportionately faster than other fitness metrics beyond the age of 50 or so, I like to emphasize shorter VO2 intervals (2-4 minutes in duration) for older athletes. This, combined with efficient weekday indoor workouts, improved his aerobic engine while also freeing up time to build his run volume and get more proficient at swimming.

Having ridden for years as a pure cyclist, Bill got into the habit of riding long on the weekends. He cherishes these rides with his mates and calls them his social therapy. Because they enhance his overall enjoyment of training, we continued to schedule these lower-intensity rides on Saturday or Sunday mornings throughout the entire training cycle. Although not the best bang-for-the-buck insofar as efficiency goes, the weekly long ride was essential, if nothing else, for Bill's well-being. Just because athletes wish to train with brutal efficiency does not mean that they have to sacrifice the reasons they got into endurance training in the first place. For Bill, this meant continuing the weekend group and coffee shop rides.

Imogene the artist

Imogene's lack of cycling strength frustrated her at first, but only fueled her desire to get better. Although it took some convincing for her to buy a power meter, once she got it, the immediate feedback and ability to track progress inspired her to be more consistent. As with most beginner cyclists, our approach was to build a foundation of cycling fitness beginning with steady riding and very soon thereafter, short intervals at tempo effort. Although the trajectory of training was similar to that of other athletes — progressive overload and a steady increase in interval duration and intensity as her fitness improved — it was clear that Imogene benefited from more engaging workouts with shorter intervals. As such, we took a more polarized training approach (higher intensity, shorter repetitions) with her, thereby inspiring her to be consistent. Cruise intervals were a great way to simulate the longer, steadier efforts most similar to triathlon racing, while still breaking up the workout.

Because Imogene wanted to do off-road triathlons, there was additional emphasis on tactics and bike handling. When the trails weren't a muddy mess, we scheduled purposeful mountain biking sessions. Since it's not realistic to prescribe targeted intervals on most trails due to their technical nature, we tried to align these sessions with her key endurance days. The result was that she spent weekdays forging her cycling fitness with high-intensity workouts and, as time allowed, combined key endurance sessions with important technical practice.

Time Hacks

-Cut out the fluff. When you have time, feel free to do various bike drills (single-leg drills, water bottle pick-ups, obstacle riding, etc.), but only if it is in addition to the meat of your workouts. On the bike, fitness tends to trump all.

-Ride indoors and always leave your bike attached to the trainer.

-Be careful, but consider shortening your warm-up. Some people need a 15 to 20-minute warm up, period. Others can get by with five minutes. You can determine your shortest possible warm-up by gradually building your power until you feel loose at tempo effort. For example, after two minutes of spinning at 55-60% of your FTP, ramp up your power by 10% every minute or so until you are comfortably spinning in Zone 3 or 4.

-Chill with the cooldown. A lot of plans prescribe 15+ minute cooldowns. Unless your physiology is exceptionally unique, you can likely get away with 5 minutes or less. But, as with the warm-up, be careful.

-Do not underestimate the value of short (30-40 minute) HIIT sessions. Have a selection of short interval workouts that you own and execute them consistently when you are time-strapped. An example could be a five minute warm-up, 10 minutes at sweetspot, 15 min of 30 seconds hard (115% FTP) 30 seconds easy; 5 minute cool-down.

-Keep it simple. When you try to do numerous different intervals at varying intensities within a workout and obsess about hitting a different cadence for each interval or part of each interval, it can get ridiculous. Unless you enjoy it, do not waste time constructing and trying to remember complicated workouts. It is a waste of mental energy. Stick to the fundamentals.

The bottom line: cut out the easy cycling and focus on a steady course of sweetspot, threshold and VO$_2$ work.

Chapter 8

The Run

How to use the most convenient discipline to your advantage

Why you should focus on it

If you are a working triathlete pressed for time, you need to embrace the run and turn it into your specialty. Running is the simplest, most convenient and time-efficient way to gain aerobic fitness. It requires minimal equipment and prep-time and can be done anywhere—even in a hotel gym at 11 PM after a business dinner. Especially for the working triathlete, focusing on developing a strong run is a worthwhile endeavor that will have an enormous impact on your overall time. For many, it is the low-hanging fruit that, if pursued, will generate the greatest return on training time invested.

Since many athletes who use the Working Triathlete training system travel often, it is common for them to execute impromptu "run blocks" in training , where all they do for a few days is run. While working with intercontinental pilots, salespeople, consultants and other individuals with travel-intensive professions, we often plan three or four days of run-focused training while they are out of town. The outcome is that these individuals enjoy fitness gains, get the opportunity to explore new cities and do not have to stress about finding a pool or a bike.

We used this approach with Bill, whose job takes him all across the country for 2-3 days each week, usually Monday through Wednesday. To balance training appropriately, we would emphasize cycling and swimming directly before and after his travel, and strictly focused on running and strength sessions during it. This allowed him to take advantage of hotel treadmills (when necessary) and weights and actually allowed him to gain run fitness faster than he might have otherwise been able to had he been distracted by low quality recumbent bikes and small pools.

Why it's important

The run is the triathlon leg during which races are won or lost. All three disciplines are important, but the run is where all your mistakes and true fitness bleed through. Many overly eager athletes with otherwise strong qualifications hit the wall in the latter stages of races. If you went too hard on the bike or messed up your nutrition, you will pay for it dearly on the run. On the flipside, if you execute an appropriate race strategy and put in the work, you will pass plenty of athletes over the last few miles.

At present, all the world champions at each triathlon distance — from sprint up to the iron distance — have a great run. Gone are the days of the uber biker putting distance between her competitors on the bike and simply hanging on during the run. If you do not have run legs, you are not going to be able to compete with the best.

Breaking down the zones and determining threshold pace

Although we covered basics in prior chapters, I want to discuss a bit further the fundamentals of run intensity zones. Similar to cycling, there are five key run intensity zones that tax similar physiological systems to corresponding cycling zones. Akin to cycling, these zones key off of your lactate threshold (Zone 4) pace, which is around the fastest pace you can maintain for an hour. The easiest way to establish your threshold is via a 30-minute field test/time trial, wherein, after a warm up, you execute an all-out 30 minute time trail by yourself on a track or other measurable surface. Your average pace over the 30-minute effort is your threshold pace and your average heart rate over the final 20 minutes is your threshold heart rate (THR).

Although it might seem that the pace you should theoretically be able to maintain for 30 minutes during a solo time trial would be faster than your lactate threshold (understood to be around the max pace you could maintain for an hour), the protocol for the field test has been empirically proven to be dead on. A 2005 study by East Carolina researchers Mcgeehee et al. showed that the results from the 30-minute test did not differ significantly from criterion that involved actually measuring the lactate threshold with instruments.

Following are the main intensity zones for running:

Running Training Zones

Zone 1

RPE: 1 to 2 **Purpose:** Active Recovery

Run Pace: Very Easy

Run % THR: <85%, **% Threshold Pace:** 130%+

Zone 2

RPE: 3-4 **Purpose:** Endurance

Run Pace: Easy

Run % THR: 85-89%, **%Threshold Pace:** 115-129%

Zone 3

RPE: 5-6 **Purpose:** Tempo

Run Pace: Moderate

Run % THR: 90-94%, **%Threshold Pace:** 105-114%

Zone 4

RPE: 7-8 **Purpose:** Threshold

Run Pace: Half Marathon to 10K

Run % THR: 95-99%, **%Threshold Pace:** 95-100%

Zone 5

RPE: 9-10 **Purpose:** VO2 Max/Aerobic capacity

Run Pace: 3K-10K

Run % THR: >100%, **%Threshold Pace>**100%

How to utilize these metrics

To demonstrate how to extrapolate training zones based on the results of a field test, assume you ran three miles during the 30-minute time trial. This equates to an average pace of 10 minutes per mile, meaning your threshold pace, or 100% of your threshold, is 10 minutes, or 600 seconds, per mile. Using this pace as the baseline, you should then refer to the chart and multiply your threshold pace by the stipulated percentages within each zone. For example, the pace for Zone 2 is 115-129% of your threshold pace. You can determine this pace by multiplying your pace per mile (10 minutes or 600 seconds) by 115% and 129%, which will give you your target pace range. For example, by multiplying 600 seconds by 115%, you get a pace of 690 seconds or 11 minutes 30 seconds per mile (600 seconds X 1.15 = 690 seconds or 11 minutes 30 seconds). For the high end of the range, multiply 600 seconds by 129%, which equals 774 seconds or 12 minutes 54 seconds per mile. In this manner, your target pace for Zone 2 is between 11:30 and 12:54 per mile.

To determine your threshold heart rate zones, you should follow the same protocol. If you averaged 150 beats per minute in the final 20 minutes of your field test, then 100% of your threshold heart rate is 150 BPM. To establish the target heart rate for each intensity zone, multiply your threshold heart rate by the percentages stipulated in that zone.

How to Structure Your Training

Although the general physiological principles governing run training are similar to cycling training, the two main differentiating factors for a busy athlete looking to maximize performance with less volume is an increase in frequency and, due to running's high impact nature, a more careful and methodical approach to integrating intensity.

Run almost every day

More so than with other disciplines, your running fitness benefits from consistency over the long term. Unlike swimming or cycling fitness, which can be maintained or expanded in as few as three workouts each week, maximizing run fitness requires more vigilance. Depending on your background and limiters, the best approach for most is to run five to six days a week, even if a couple of those runs are short (e.g., 15 to 20-minute brick workouts). With shorter, more frequent workouts, you can increase overall volume with less stress on the body. The high-impact nature of longer runs, especially exacerbated by the inevitable breakdown of form as duration increases, very often leads to injury. So be smart: run frequently, listen to your body, but don't destroy yourself, as so many do, obsessing about maximizing the duration of your long run.

Because frequency is so important, the majority of your runs should be in the 30 to 60 minute range at Zone 2 intensity. This allows for solid stimulus with limited recovery costs. Day in and day out, Zone 3 runs should be avoided since they offer poor benefit relative to cost. Left to their own devices, many athletes naturally fall into Zone 3 pace, which carries with it higher recovery costs and little physiological benefit in excess of Zone 2 efforts. Apart from race pace efforts or brief builds or pick-ups within longer runs, you should focus on emphasizing Zone 2, 4 and occasionally Zone 5 efforts; however, adding intensity needs to be done intelligently and you should not jeopardize frequency in order to accomplish long, high-cost, high-intensity sessions.

How to intelligently incorporate intensity

Although you can integrate high-intensity cycling sessions fairly soon in a macrocycle, you should be more cautious when incorporating harder running workouts. Especially for newer runners, older athletes, and/or those with muscle imbalances or flexibility issues, the likelihood of eventual injury is high. Until you accomplish a solid base of easy miles to strengthen your hard and soft tissue to withstand steady running, you should not engage in high-volume, aerobic capacity or upper threshold workouts.

If run training is not tailored to the individual, injury is almost certain. For example, if we compare Maximus, who had no run background when he started working with us, to Kim, who ran a few times each week for years, it is clear that their run schedule needed to be different. For Maximus, the emphasis was gradually building up mileage with a keen eye on avoiding injury. For Kim, we were able to begin at a higher volume and harness her run ability and resiliency and integrate slightly higher intensity sessions sooner.

For most triathletes, the run emphasis throughout the majority of the General Preparation Subphase should be on developing general aerobic fitness and durability — predominately through easier Zone 2 running. These easier efforts should be supplemented by fairly short, intense efforts in the form of hills, strides and pick-ups in order to stay in touch with the neuromuscular demands of faster running. As the Preparation Phase advances and your body acclimates to the high-impact demand of running, you can then begin to execute a mix of threshold and VO2-focused (Zone 4-5) workouts as well as race pace efforts; though, relative to cycling, the frequency and duration of harder interval sessions should be lower.

Different coaches have different philosophies, but unless someone has a running background, is running at least 20 miles a week, or has proven to have a sturdy body (e.g., is a former athlete in a running intensive sport like soccer or football), I usually do not prescribe long intervals faster than 5K pace. Even then, the majority of mileage is easy. There are plenty of low-risk gains to be had by simply increasing volume in the form of persistent, shorter Zone 2 efforts.

Irrespective of the risks, if you intelligently incorporate specific high-intensity running into your training plan, you should be able to avoid injury and maintain a high level of performance. The key is being conservative and gradually increasing the load. This means emphasizing hill workouts and pick-ups early in the macrocycle and, only later on, integrating high-duration, high-intensity running in the form of tempo runs, intervals and long runs.

Types of high-intensity running

Hills

Hills are advantageous early in the training cycle for building strength, maximizing muscle recruitment and improving coordination between muscle groups. Because you are running up an incline, there is less vertical oscillation at high intensity and therefore less pounding. For beginning hill work, I prescribe that athletes find a long hill with a 4-8% grade or utilize a treadmill with an adjustable gradient. The athlete should perform 4-8 X 45 seconds intervals up the hill at a strong but not maximum effort with an easy recovery jog back down the hill. As fitness improves, the duration and number of intervals should increase. Later in the training cycle, hill workouts are typically replaced with more conventional interval sessions, though some hill training can still be beneficial and even necessary if the target race is hilly. For certain athletes with a greater propensity for injury (such as older or new runners like Bill and Maximus), or while training for hilly races, it makes sense to do traditional interval workouts at incline on a treadmill in order to achieve a high-intensity stimulus with less impact.

Strides

Another form of high-intensity running that should be implemented year-round and before every race or hard workout is strides. These are short build ups wherein you steadily accelerate to 90-95% of your sprint speed over 40 to 100 meters while focusing on running tall, pumping your arms, lifting your knees and maintaining good form. Performing four to eight of these strides a few times a week is beneficial for maintaining and fostering strong running mechanics. By executing these, you will remain in touch with the neurological demands of faster running and will avoid becoming an athlete whose one gear is a slow plod.

Pick-Ups

Another low-stress way to integrate faster running into your schedule is via pick-ups, which are short increases in pace interspersed throughout a supporting or key endurance session. Pick-ups usually last 1-4 minutes and are typically between 10K and marathon pace. The goal of these is not necessarily to tax the cardiorespiratory system or generate lactate — you should not be huffing and puffing after each pick-up. The purpose is similar to that of strides: i.e., form and neuromuscular maintenance. An example of a set of pick-ups would be 4X1:30 at threshold pace with 2 minutes of recovery in the middle of a 45-minute supporting run.

Integrating core high-intensity sessions

Although there is much to be said for emphasizing frequent easy runs, if you want to maximize your potential, you need to incorporate core high-intensity sessions. To be clear, those at the pointy end of the field need to run fast and run often. Especially for the more competitive athletes we coach (former collegiate runners, national/world qualifiers, etc.), we schedule one to two higher intensity sessions each week throughout the training cycle. But even average and below-average triathletes can and should integrate harder running. The key, no matter your fitness, is intelligently executing key intensity workouts that align with your experience, physical resiliency and racing goals.

For triathlons, run distances range from a couple kilometers up to the marathon, and the structure of key intensity sessions should vary depending upon which race distance you are training for; however, you may be surprised that the training across distances is more similar than different. With the exception of the unique metabolic demands that you will face in long course racing, the performance of the physiological systems that you will use in every distance from sprint triathlons up to the iron distance are forged in the same manner.

At the risk of oversimplifying, the essential training goals for all distances should be the same: to maximize your lactate threshold, running economy and VO2 max. If you improve these, you will be able to race faster and your cruise or "all-day-pace" will increase in relative proportion to the strength of these metrics. There are additional considerations for long course, such as development of general endurance and ability to withstand the deep muscular fatigue and trauma that arises when the duration of exercise is exceptionally long, but the fundamentals are the same. Apart from certain race-specific workouts (i.e., high-duration sessions in the case for iron-distance race preparation; high intensity bricks for sprint distance, etc.), run training for sprint triathlons and iron distance races are quite similar, with tempo/threshold runs and various interval workouts comprising the meat of high-intensity run training.

Threshold/Tempo

Threshold or tempo runs are sessions where you run at approximately your lactate threshold, or Zone 4 pace. The purpose is to teach the body to efficiently clear lactate, which will allow you to run at a higher intensity before having to slow down.

The most common or classic threshold workout is a 20 to 30-minute tempo run wherein you run at a comfortably hard pace for ~20-30 minutes. This duration is long enough to generate a strong stimulus without producing deep fatigue and it is common to do two of these in a single session (e.g. 2X2 miles, 2X20 minutes, etc.). Some coaches may prescribe "tempo runs" of up to 60 continuous minutes in duration, but these are typically run well below threshold pace and deliver a slightly different physiological and psychological benefit.

Other variations of workouts predominately run around threshold pace include cruise intervals, which are longish (800 meters to 2 miles) intervals at approximately Zone 4 pace or slightly faster with very short rest (30-60 seconds). Cruise intervals deliver a stimulus very similar to classic tempo runs but are mentally easier due to the rest periods. Beginners can especially benefit from cruise intervals because of the brief break between intervals and are more likely to maintain proper form and intensity.

Aside from hill workouts, threshold running should be one of the first higher-intensity sessions you introduce within a macrocycle. Because they are slightly less grueling than workouts focused on Zone 5 intensities, they can be incorporated in varying fashion throughout the Preparation and Competitive phases of training.

Intervals

The other important category of high-intensity running is interval work near aerobic capacity, which is usually composed of faster-paced intervals in upper Zone 4 and 5. These are repeats of one to eight minutes (~400-2000 meters) done at 3K-10K race pace and separated by rest intervals that are typically 50%-100% of the interval duration. For example, if you are doing 400-meter repeats in 70 seconds, your recovery interval should be 35 to 70 seconds.

One of the cornerstone VO2/aerobic capacity interval workouts are 800-meter repeats completed at 5K race pace. A beginner should start with a session of four intervals separated by rest intervals of equal duration. As fitness improves, the number of intervals should increase while rest decreases.

VO2 intervals have their place in training for all triathlon distances, even iron distance. Although you should not come close to Zone 5 intensity in long course racing, by integrating higher intensity into your training, you raise your aerobic ceiling and spur cardiorespiratory fitness adaptations that can only be realized via hard running, such as increases in the size and number of mitochondria and a markedly increased ability to process oxygen. As I cautioned previously, however, hard intervals have a high recovery cost and should be approached cautiously. You should pay special attention to form when doing them and focus intently on adequate recovery by practicing good nutrition, getting enough rest and not engaging in hard exercise the subsequent day.

Long/Key Endurance Runs

The final important workout in the runner's arsenal is the long run or key endurance session. Although of secondary importance to overall volume and frequency, long runs, or runs of a duration substantially longer than your key intensity and supporting sessions, are important for inducing metabolic adaptations (burning more fat as fuel) and teaching the body to cope with the deep muscular trauma and fatigue of racing. For long course races, runs over 90 minutes are essential and most would be served well with a long run peaking at approximately two hours. I have found that there is little to no additional physiological benefit beyond that duration due to recovery. Granted, there may be worthwhile psychological benefits for certain athletes beyond two hours, so consideration of individualized needs is important.

The goal race will determine the frequency and length of the long run. If a busy athlete is solely focused on sprint triathlons, the necessity of a long run over eight miles might not be defensible. The cost does not justify the benefit for such a short race and a time-strapped athlete could be better served integrating more intensity and emphasizing recovery. For Olympic through long course racing, however, the necessity and usefulness of a long endurance focused session increases. In most cases, due to the difficulty working athletes face trying to recover from long runs, I find that limiting the frequency to once every ten days is superior to cramming in a progressively lengthier long run every week.

Good running form

Although dramatically altering your form or forcing a style that is not conducive to your build is not advisable, there are certain universal traits of good running form that will allow you to run faster and with less stress on your body.

Breathing: You should aim to get plenty of air while running. Breathe through both your mouth and nose by taking deep belly breaths. Your stomach should expand and contract with each breath.

Posture: You should run tall with your spine and neck in alignment. A slight forward lean is optimal. Your shoulders should be down (not scrunched) and your neck, shoulders and hands should be relaxed. Act as if you are holding a butterfly in each hand and don't want to crush them. Tension is not efficient.

Arm carriage: Your arms should be bent at approximately 90 degrees and should pump forward and backward. Make sure they do not swing across over your center line.

Stride: Make sure that your foot falls beneath your center of gravity. Most peoples' feet hit the ground too far in front of them, leading to a breaking effect that destroys momentum and causes injury. Strive to be light on your feet and experiment with a faster cadence. A stride rate of 180 foot falls per minute is often described as ideal, but everyone is different.

Putting it all together

Now that you have a basic understanding of the terms and rationale behind the Working Triathlete approach to run training, let's concisely hone in on how you might integrate it over a full training cycle.

Preparation Phase (usually 8-16 weeks)

In the General Preparation Subphase, focus on running 5-6 times per week at Zone 2 intensity. Incorporate short 1 to 3-minute sub-threshold pick-ups into a couple of your weekly supporting runs and do strides a few times a week.

After a couple weeks of easy running, gradually integrate hill running to build strength. As the General Preparation Phase continues, maintain frequency. Once your body can withstand a decently high training volume (~20+ miles per week), you can begin integrating higher intensity running in the form of threshold and VO2 workouts. Most should aim for one key intensity session and one key endurance session each week. If you are focusing on long course, the importance of the key endurance session should be emphasized, but remember to never sacrifice frequency and consistency for occasional big days.

In the Specific Preparation Subphase, you should continue building your training load and focus on developing race-specific fitness. For sprint triathlon training, this means emphasizing VO2 work (e.g. 6X800 at 5K pace; 12X400 at 3K pace; etc.) and for the iron distance, getting comfortable running for 2+ hours.

Competition Phase (usually 6-10 weeks)

In the Pre-Competition Subphase you should continue emphasizing race-specific work without jeopardizing frequency. Like with cycling training, the load may plateau or decrease in anticipation of a series of races; however, especially early on, assuming you have been adhering to the Working Triathlete training approach, you will not and should not need to cut your training load by a substantial amount.

As the core Competition Subphase begins, you need to focus on balancing racing and recovery with fitness maintenance. Continue running 5-6 times per week while prioritizing recovery. Keep the training polarized. It is common to get injured in this phase as the overall impact of high-intensity sessions begins to take their toll on the body, so make sure you maintain good form, continue auxiliary strength training and recover well. Like with cycling, your taper should commence approximately two weeks prior to your A-race with a gradual reduction in volume but with a continued emphasis on short Zone 4-5 efforts to keep the central nervous system primed.

Transition Phase (usually 2-4 weeks)

As described in prior chapters, after your final race, you should engage in a couple of weeks of rest or active recovery.

How Maximus, Kim, Bill and Imogene successfully approached run training

Maximus the magnificent swimmer

For people like Maximus who enter triathlon with prior experience in swimming, cycling rowing or some other endurance sport—the aerobic engine often does not often match the physical durability of the tendons, ligaments and joints. As a life-long swimmer, Maximus had very flexible ankles that immediately started bothering him, shortly followed by shin splints and mild knee pain. To manage, we had him run on treadmills (slightly lower-impact than running on concrete), strategically scheduled pool running sessions and were careful not to integrate intensity too soon. We also avoided run-bike brick workouts to avoid having him run with poor, injury-inducing form. After two months of pure Z2 running (plus strides), we increased the average duration of his run sessions and began integrating tempo efforts. As his iron distance race approached, we also focused on extending the duration of his key endurance sessions to ensure that he had the muscular resilience and psychological strength and confidence to complete the marathon, which he accomplished without walking a step (except through the aid stations, where it is important to focus on getting in appropriate nutrition).

Kim the corporate executive

Kim had a textbook run build throughout her first macrocycle with us, beginning with steady Z2 runs, hills and pick-ups and then moving to threshold and interval sessions. Since she was not prone to running injuries, she was able to execute a quality key intensity and key endurance session weekly. Most of her weekday runs were brick workouts that, although short, delivered substantial weekly volume. This approach allowed her to consistently run people down at the end of her races and achieve top-5 age group run splits at regional races.

Bill the older uber biker

Our approach to run training with Bill mirrored Maximus's, although we were particularly cautious in building volume. Older athletes often struggle to stay injury free while running, so being conservative with load and emphasizing good running mechanics was paramount. Bill never saw the same overall volume or intensity as Maximus, Kim or Imogene, but he ran just as frequently, which allowed him to avoid injury while maximizing fitness gains. These short but frequent runs allowed him to put down very good run splits, proving that consistency with running trumps all.

Imogene the artist

As a recreational runner, Imogene took to running naturally and enjoyed it. Nevertheless, her form when she started with us was lacking and she struggled with knee pain. To combat this, we emphasized developing strong biomechanics, especially in the form of strides, building core strength, and were careful integrating intensity or building volume too quickly. With our careful approach, her physical resiliency and fitness improved dramatically. Because one of her goals was to complete an off-road triathlon, we made sure she ran plenty of miles on trails so as to develop ankle strength and confidence running on rugged terrain. Like Kim, she was able to adhere to the typical Working Triathlete approach to run training and has consistently finished among the top athletes in her age group.

Six pillars of run training:

-Run 5-6 times each week.

-Keep most of your runs short: 30-60 minutes in Zone 2 and focus on good form.

-Keep your easy days easy so that you can nail your key sessions.

-Do strides often and with great technique.

-When building intensity, begin with hills, then move to threshold workouts and finally VO2 workouts.

-Long runs are important, but do not overemphasize their importance to the detriment of overall consistency.

Chapter 9

Strength Training

How to reap the benefits of being strong

Endurance athletes often get a rap for being skinny. In fact, many avoid the weight room for fear of getting too bulky, which is a mistake. To be certain, there is some merit to being lean and not carrying superfluous mass. However, assuming you do not go overboard by lifting heavy weights every day, eating absurd quantities of food and cutting out most of your endurance training, you will not gain pounds of stringy muscle mass (sorry wannabe Arnolds). It simply does not work that way. You will, however, get stronger and experience other myriad benefits that make strength training a worthwhile endeavor even for busy working athletes.

The purpose of strength training

The purpose of strength training for performance-oriented triathletes is different than for body builders and power lifters. Rather than getting large or moving as much weight as possible, the goal is to build functional strength that will translate into greater and more coordinated power and superior form and joint stability, which can boost exercise economy and prevent injury. Quite simply, a good strength training program can make you faster and more durable.

Power=Speed

Endurance sports require strength. Yes, carrying extra weight, even in the form of muscle, can detrimentally impact performance; however, you need to be able to generate enough force to actually go fast. This does not mean that you need to gain a lot of muscle mass — the goal is to be strong relative to your weight. Especially for swimming and cycling, the strength required to propel your body forward requires substantial muscular power. The stronger you are, the smaller the percentage of overall max power you will have to exert in order to maintain a given pace. You will also be better able to maintain your form in the latter stages of a race when muscle fatigue sets in, better positioning yourself for the final kick.

According to a study published in 2015 by Damasceno, et al., "a strength training program offers a potent stimulus to counteract fatigue during the last parts of a 10-km running race, resulting in an improved overall running performance." The study separated a group of 18 endurance runners into a strength training group or control group and had the strength training group engage in an 8-week strength training program. In addition to experiencing a higher magnitude of improvement in a drop jump and peak treadmill speed test, the strength group improved their 10-km running performance by 2.5% versus -.07% for the control group.

Strength training can improve form and exercise economy

Just as being stronger can improve absolute power output during endurance training and racing, so too can it improve running economy, or the amount of oxygen you consume at a given pace relative to your body weight. Being stronger allows you to recruit the correct muscles for an optimized stride, allowing you to run with superior and efficient form for a longer period of time. As evidence, a 2008 study by Storen et al. separated a group of runners into two groups: one of which executed a tri-weekly strength routine of half squats while the other (control group) continued their normal endurance training regimen. After eight weeks, the strength group improved running economy by 5% and time to exhaustion at maximal aerobic speed by 21.3%. The control group experienced no changes from pre- to post-values in these parameters.

Strength training can prevent injury

Apart from impacting exercise economy, improper form resulting from weak or imbalanced muscles can lead to excess load on joints, ligaments and tendons — all of which are main factors contributing to overuse injuries. For example, due to weak glutes, hips and quadriceps, many peoples' knees collapse inward when running or squatting, leading to PFS (knee) and IT Band pain. Strengthening these weak muscles can facilitate proper form, allowing you to exercise more efficiently and with a lower propensity for developing overuse injuries.

Over the years we have found that women especially benefit from working on strengthening hips and quads due to their larger Q-angle (angle at which femur meets the tibia), which often leads to lateral force on their knees when they run. For example, when we started working with Imogene, she could not do a single squat without her knees collapsing inward. This led to a host of biomechanical issues, including pronation and knee pain when she ran long distances. By focusing on increasing strength with an emphasis on core stability work (especially single leg squats, leg raises and bridges), we were able to improve her stride, running economy and prevent injury.

But strength training does not just improve biomechanics and coordination; it literally makes your body more durable. According to a study published in Sports Medicine, "Research indicates that resistance training promotes growth and/or increases in the strength of ligaments, tendons, tendon to bone and ligament to bone junction strength, joint cartilage and the connective tissue sheaths within muscle. Studies involving humans and animal models also demonstrate resistance training can cause increased bone mineral content and therefore may aid in prevention of skeletal injuries. Investigations to date suggest resistance training can aid in injury prevention. The incidence of various types of overuse injuries, such as swimmers shoulder and tennis elbow, may be reduced by the performance of sport and/or motion specific resistance training activities" (Fleck 1986).

You will stay leaner, recover better and maintain fitness

Apart from the biomechanical benefits, strength training delivers a host of other physiological benefits that can boost performance, including improved body composition and hormone levels.

When you lift weights, you are obviously burning calories to perform the movements, but you are also building metabolically active muscle tissue that will boost your baseline metabolic rate, allowing you to consistently burn more calories. This makes it easier to maintain appropriate body composition, which is essential for strong performance.

Similarly, lifting heavy weights — especially via compound movements wherein you utilize large muscle groups — can spur the release of testosterone and other hormones essential for proper recovery. This is beneficial for endurance athletes since aerobic training can inhibit endocrine function and lower testosterone levels. By focusing on key core lifts like squats and dead lifts, you can counteract this reduction, leading to better training and recovery.

A note for older athletes

The benefits of strength training are especially magnified as you age. Although we all may be able to get away with minimal strength training and eating whatever we want when we are young, as we get older our muscle mass and strength naturally decreases. Lifting weights can stall or reverse this trend, allowing you to maintain muscle mass and continue generating the power that will enable you to execute key workouts and race well.

The benefits of lifting weights were especially evident when we began working with Bill, who, at the age of 59, never adhered to a serious strength training regimen. Although he was by no means fat, it was clear that his performance could improve if he increased his lean muscle mass and power. To address this, we had him perform two full-body strength training sessions each week after his swims. The result was that after a few months his body fat dropped a few percentage points, his strength improved and he simply felt better. His wife also preferred the slightly less doughy look.

A strength training program for the time-strapped athlete

Integrating an effective strength training routine does not require a significant time commitment. For most athletes, I recommend at least one full-body strength session each week along with shorter sessions focused on auxiliary exercises (i.e. glute/hip stability, etc.). Older athletes like Bill should strive for two full-body strength sessions in addition to shorter auxiliary exercise sessions. Fortunately, these full-body workouts can be completed in as little as 30 minutes if you focus on the most important and effective movements.

Similarly to other disciplines, the Working Triathlete approach to strength training is grounded in reaping maximum benefit with minimal time investment. This means focusing only on lifts and exercises that deliver the greatest and most efficient strength gains pertinent to triathlon training and racing.

Although there are thousands of possible exercises, you can capture nearly all potential strength benefits by executing what I like to refer to as the six Core Lifts, which are dead lifts, squats, bench press, pull ups/pull downs, barbell rows and military press. Although we prescribe workouts with additional exercises, these movements are the focal point of the Working Triathlete strength training routine and sessions composed of them are referred to as the Core Strength Workouts (see below for more detail). All six lifts can be performed in a single session and are brutally efficient for building full-body strength and power since they engage large muscle groups and require the utilization of multiple joints to perform. In addition to the Core Strength Workout, you should also perform auxiliary exercises that focus on addressing muscle weaknesses and imbalances, though these are secondary to the Core Strength Workout and can be done at convenient times throughout the week as time allows.

111

Core Strength Session

All athletes should strive to do at least one Core Strength Session each week up to the Competition Subphase or through the Build Period. Older athletes should strive for two sessions per week through these phases.

Core Strength Workout Structure: do three sets of 5-15 repetitions of each of the Core Lifts as described below. Make sure you execute each repetition with proper form (seek the assistance of an experienced and certified personal trainer to ensure proper form). If you are new to strength training, start with lighter weight and more repetitions. As you get stronger and more comfortable, lower the number of repetitions and increase the weight.

-**Dead Lifts:** 3 Sets of 5-15 Repetitions

-**Squats:** 3 Sets of 5-15 Repetitions

-**Bench Press** (dumbbell or barbell on flat or incline benches): 3 Sets of 8-15 Repetitions

-**Pull-ups or pull-downs:** 3 Sets of 5-15 Repetitions

-**Barbell Rows:** 3 Sets of 8-15 Repetitions

-**Military Press:** 3 Sets of 8-15 Repetitions.

Auxiliary Exercise Session

In addition to the Core Strength Workout, you should complete twice-weekly auxiliary exercise sessions. You can squeeze these in at any point within the day (i.e., when you wake up, in your hotel room, over lunch, etc.), or even before or after your Core Strength workout.

Auxiliary exercises focus on smaller muscle groups and, especially for endurance athletes, are often used to address muscle imbalances or under-performing muscles, including hip abductors and adductors, glutes, or specific parts of your quadriceps group. These muscles are responsible for proper alignment and stabilizing your core.

Auxiliary Strength Workout Structure

Complete two sets of each exercise as described below. If you are a beginner, keep the sets shorter and gradually increase the number of repetitions or duration as you gain strength. Focus on slow, controlled movements. Brief descriptions of each exercise are below:

-**Bridges (unilateral):** 2 Sets of 10-20 Repetitions per leg

-**Clam Shell:** 2 Sets of 10-20 Repetitions per leg

-**Side Plank Leg Raises:** 2 Sets of 10-20 Repetitions

-**Side-Lying Hip Adduction:** 2 Sets of 10-20 Repetitions

-**Straight Leg Lifts:** 2 Sets of 10-20 Repetitions

-**Single Leg Squats:** 2 Sets of 10-20 Repetitions

-**Bird Dog:** 2 Sets of 10-20 Repetitions

-**Russian Twist:** 2 Sets Lasting 30-60 Seconds

-**Flutter Kicks:** 2 Sets Lasting 30-60 Seconds

-**Plank:** 2 Sets Lasting 30-60 Seconds

Bridges: Lie on your back with your right leg bent at the knee and your right foot flat on the ground. The left leg should be straight. Press down with your right foot by engaging your glute and lift your hip and straight leg off the ground. Make sure your left leg, hips and torso are in a straight line. Only your upper back, head and foot should be on the ground. Hold this position for three seconds and slowly lower your hips down again to the starting position. This is one repetition for the right leg.

Clam Shell: Lie on your side with your legs on top of one another and bent at the knee at a 45 degree angle. Make sure that your hips and shoulders are aligned in one straight line and do not arch your back or strain your neck .While keeping the sides of your feet together, lift your top knee so that it is parallel to your hip. Lower your knee back to the starting position. This is one repetition for one leg.

Side Plank Leg Lift: Place your right elbow and forearm on the ground and straighten your legs, keeping your core lifted off the ground and balanced on the outside edge of your right foot. Slowly lift your left leg upward to slightly above your hip, then slowly lower it back down. This is one repetition for the left leg.

Side-Lying Hip Adduction: Lie on your right side with your legs straight but with your right foot just in front of your left. Slowly raise your right leg upward until you feel tension in your groin. Slowly lower it back down. This is one repetition for your right leg.

Straight Leg Lifts: Lie on your back with your legs straight. Lift one leg keeping it straight until it creates a 45-degree angle with the ground. Slowly lower it back down to the starting position. This is one repetition for one leg. As a variation, lie on your side and lift your leg upward until you feel tension in your outer hip. You should use ankle weights to increase difficulty.

Single Leg Squat: Stand with one foot on the ground. Slowly bend your leg, lowering yourself until your femur is parallel to the ground. Pause for one second and slowly raise yourself back to the starting position. Keep your back straight throughout the whole movement and keep weight on your heel. This is one repetition for one leg.

Bird Dog: Kneel on the ground with your knees and hands on the ground. Raise your right arm and left leg so that both are parallel to the ground. Slowly lower them back to the starting position. This is one repetition for one side of your body.

Russian Twist: Sit with your torso leaning back at a 45-degree angle with your knees bent and feet off the ground. Twist your torso and touch the ground on either side of your body. Continue doing this, alternating sides. You can hold a dumbbell or medicine ball for extra weight and stimulus.

Flutter Kicks: Lie down on your back with your legs straight. Lift your feet off the ground just a few inches and kick your legs similarly to the way you do in swimming, keeping your legs straight and only moving them up and down a few inches to ignite your lower abs.

Plank: Lie face-down, balancing on your forearms with your toes on the ground and your core engaged and your legs, spine and neck in alignment. Hold this position while maintaining a straight back.

Part 3

The Plans

Chapter 10

Training Plans

Comprehensive General Prep for Olympic/Half-Iron and Race Specific Half Iron Plans

The training plans offered in this book are meant to serve as guides for executing training. You can do every workout precisely as described in the order herein and be successful, but you should take the liberty to adjust the plan a bit to suit your lifestyle. The point of Working Triathlete is to create a framework for training that you can adapt to fit your busy life. There is, however, a careful rationale to the sequence within and between microcycles, so the better you adhere to the plan as laid out, the higher your likelihood of success. You can find additional and more detailed training plans at www.workingtriathlete.com

As written, the plans assume that athletes wish to be competitive and that they have a basic foundation of endurance fitness — i.e., they can run at least 50 minutes, cycle at least 1.5 hours and easily swim 1000 yards without stopping. If you cannot do that, you should extend the General Preparation Phase on the front end by engaging in a mesocycle of Zone 2 endurance work until you have the capacity to complete these prerequisites.

Plan Structure

There are two different plans laid out in this book: a 12-week General Preparation/Base Plan which can be used for all distances, and a 12-week Half Iron Race Specific Plan that covers the time period from the Specific Preparation Subphase up through the race (i.e., the final 12 weeks leading up to the race). If you are looking for a comprehensive Half Iron Plan, you should stack the 12-week General Preparation Plan with the 12-week Race Specific Plan.

If you are inexperienced or wish to extend the General Preparation Plan, you can extend it for as long as you see fit so long as you do not dramatically alter the training load. Alternatively, if you are time-strapped, you can use the 12-Week General Preparation Plan as your main training plan for Sprint and Olympic distance races. The volume and intensity is sufficient to get you to the finish line.

Each week prescribes key intensity and endurance sessions within each discipline. These sessions are the most important sessions of each week and every effort should be made to execute these. As a rule, key intensity sessions are separated by at least one day and are intended to be accomplished early in the week. The key endurance sessions (long rides/runs) are usually placed on the weekends for convenience.

Interpreting Workouts

For your own convenience and to simplify as much as possible, the workouts are stripped down to their essential components. There is no fluff. As you are reading, you may encounter the following short hand:

Key I or Key E: Key Intensity or Key Endurance session

Cadence: Instructs you to vary cadence. For cycling, low cadence is 40-60 RPMs and high cadence is over 100 RPMs. Always follow low-cadence work with high-cadence work. A common example is one minute of low-cadence work followed by one minute of high-cadence.

(SST) or Upper Z3: Refers to maintaining intensity in the sweetspot zone or at sweetspot intensity, which is 85-93% of FTP, or just below threshold intensity.

OTB: Refers to a run "Off the Bike."

PUs or Pick-Ups: Refers to short increases in intensity or pace, usually to a Zone 3 or 4 effort.

Rec or Recovery or Rest Interval or (#): Refers to the amount of recovery time between intervals. For VO2 intervals, target a recovery time equal to or slightly less than the interval duration. For threshold efforts, target a smaller fraction of time, typically one to five minutes. As an example ,3X10 Z4 (5) would mean three, ten minute intervals at Zone 4 intensity with five minutes of rest between each.

Examples: Although most workouts are straightforward, some can seem complicated. For example, if a cycling workout stipulates 50: Cad: 8X(2 low, 2 high) SST (2), it is instructing you to do 8 intervals of 2 minutes at a low cadence and 2 minutes at a high cadence (so each interval totals four minutes), with two minute recoveries. The "50" indicates the total duration of the workout including warm up and cool down.

Other considerations: You should warm up at least 5-15 minutes before each workout, and cool down for a similar duration as time allows.

Swim Workouts

Due to space constraints, the structure of swim workouts are not included in the chart; however, the type of workout, either Key Intensity (Muscular Endurance), Key Endurance (General Endurance) or form, is noted.

For simplicity and efficacy, each swim workout should follow the same structure: warm-up, pre-set, main-set and cool-down. The warm-up, pre-set, and cool-down can be structured the same from workout to workout (though you should switch drill types in the pre-set). The main-set will change.

For the warm-up, you should swim easily for 5-10 minutes. After that you should transition immediately into a pre-set composed of drills interspersed with easy swimming. You then execute the main-set, which is the meat of the workout (examples of which are below). You should then finish with a 100-300 yard/meter pull as a cool-down. If you are time-strapped, emphasize the main-set and trim or eliminate the other parts of the workout.

Following is a guide for your swim sessions. As you can see, the warm-up, pre-set and cool-downs are similar. For the main-set, you should identify what your prescribed workout type is (key intensity, key endurance, or form) and choose a set to reflect the goal. You can cycle through these or modify them for variety and/or to suit your fitness level.

Warm-Up

5-10 minutes of easy swimming

Pre-Set

2-3X150 yards/meters

-50 Kick Drill (choice — with or without fins or a kickboard, on your back, on your side, etc.)

-50 Drill (choice — single arm freestyle, catch-up, fist, finger-tip, scull, etc.)

-50 easy swim

Main-Set (choose one based on the prescribed type of workout. All can be shortened or lengthened depending on your fitness)

Key Intensity/Muscular Endurance (Short Intervals, High Intensity, Z4-5)

#1 20X50 Z4-5 (20)

#2 10X100 Z4 (20)

#3 4X (25-50-75-100) Z4-5 (20)

#4 12X25, 8X50 Z4-5 (10-20)

#5 15X75 Z4-5 (10-20)

#6 8X150 Z4 (20)

#7 6X200 Z4 (20)

Key Endurance/General Endurance (Long Intervals, Lower Intensity, Z2-4)

#1 8X200 Z3 (10)

#2 500-400-300-200-100 Z3-4 (20-30)

#3 4X400 Z3 (30)

#4 4X300 Z3-4 (30)

#5 1X400, 4X200, 1X400 pull, Z3 (30)

#6 2X (400, 200, 100) Z3-4 (30)

#7 Open Water (or simulation), continuous or with breaks as needed, 1000-4000 yards/meters

Form:

#1 5X (50 catch-up, 50 fist, 50 freestyle, 50 single arm) Z2-3 (30)

#2 Any workout, sight every length

120

#3 4X300 Z2-3 (30) with a snorkel

#4 10X100 or 5X200 Z3-4 (30) striving to maximize distance per stroke every other lap

#5 Stroke rate: 6X150 Z3 (30) alternate between catch up, zipper and natural freestyle every lap

Cool-Down

Swim with pull buoy for 100-300 yards focusing on a good catch

For additional and more detailed swim workouts, consider downloading a plan from www.workingtriathlete.com

catch up - arms meet out front, thumbs interlock

Zipper - arm/hand/thumb runs up body

finger tip - drag finger tips across top of water

12-Week General Preparation

For Sprint, Olympic and Half Iron Distances

The following 12-Week General Preparation Plan will prepare your body for the rigors of racing and hard training. You can race reasonably competitively off of the fitness generated by adhering to this 12-week plan, though its main purpose is to serve as the first half of a comprehensive 24-week macrocycle culminating in an A-Race.

A few highlights:

-The plan is structured so that you can adjust it to the time you have available, with optional workouts and opportunities to extend the duration.

-The plan is designed in four-week mesocycles, with three build weeks and one recovery week in which fatigue is unloaded.

-The schedule assumes you have an endurance background. If you are a pure beginner, execute a base of Z2 work before tackling the plan.

12-Week General Prep/Base Phase

Week		MON	TUE	WED	THU	FRI	SAT	SUN
1	AM	Form Swim: 30-60 Z2-3	Key Bike I: 40: 2X10 SST (3)	Key Swim I: 30: Z3-Z4	Bike: 40: Middle 15 SST	Key Swim E: 40-60 Z2-3	Key Bike E: 60: Middle 20 SST	Key Run E:40: Z2. 4X1 Z3-4 PUs
	PM	Optional Strength: 30	Run: 30: Z2	Run: 30: Z2 + Strides	Strength: 30	Run: 35: Z2 + Strides	Run: 20 min Brick OTB	
2	AM	Optional Swim: 30-60 Z2-3, Form	Key Bike I: 45: 4X3 Z5 (3)	Key Swim I: 30: Z3-Z4	Bike: 45: 8X1 Z5 (1)	Key Swim E: 40-60: Z2-3	Key Bike E: 65: 3X10 SST (3)	Key Run E:45 Z2 + Strides
	PM	Optional Strength: 30	Run: 35: Z2	Run: 30: Z2 + Strides	Strength: 30	Run: 35: Z2, 4X1 min Z4	Run: 20 min Brick OTB	
3	AM	Optional Swim: 30-60: Z2-3, Form	Key Bike I: 45: Middle 15 Z4	Key Swim I: 30: Z3-4	Bike: 45: Cadence. 8X (2 low, 1 high) Z3 (3)	Key Swim E: 40-60 Z2-3	Key Bike E: 65: Middle 30 SST	Key Run E+I:50: Z2 w/ Hills 6X45 sec Z5 (2)
	PM	Optional Strength: 30	Run: 35: Z2	Run: 35: Z2 + strides	Strength: 30	Run: 35: Z2 + Strides	Run: 20 min Brick OTB	
4	AM	Optional Swim: 30-60 Z2-3, Form	Key Bike I: 45: 4X5 Z4, (2)	Key Swim I: 30: Z3-Z4	Bike: 45: 2X10 SST, (2)	Key Swim E: 40-60: Z2-3	Key Bike E: 60: 20 min SST, 20 min, Mid Z3 (3)	Key Run E+I: 50 Z2. 4X1:30 Z4 (2)
	PM	Optional Strength: 30	Run: 30: Z2	Run: 30: Z2 + Strides	Strength: 30	Run: 35: Z2 + strides	Run: 20 min Brick OTB	
5	AM	Optional Swim: 30-60: Z2-3, Form	Key Bike I: 60: 2X15 Z4, (5)	Key Swim I: 40: Z3	Bike: 45: 6X1 Z5 (1), 20 Mid Z3	Key Swim E: 40-60 Z2-3	Key Bike E: 70: 1X10 Z3, 2X10 Z4, (4)	Key Run E+I: 60: Z2 w/ 4X2 min Z3-4 PUs
	PM	Optional Strength: 30	Run: 35: Z2	Run: 40: Z2 + strides	Strength: 30	Run: 45: Z2 + Strides	Run: 20 min Brick OTB	
6	AM	Optional Swim: 30-60 Z2-3, Form	Key Bike I: 60: 6X5 Z4 (2)	Key Swim I: 40: Z3-Z4	Bike: 50: Cad: 8X (2 min low, 2 min high) SST(2)	Key Swim E: 40-60: Z2-3	Key Bike E: 75: 4X10 SST (4)	Key Run E+I: 60: Z2-4 Hills 6X60 Z5 (2)
	PM	Optional Strength: 30	Run: 35: Z2	Run: 40: Z2 + Strides	Strength: 30	Run: 45: Z2 + strides	Run: 20 min Brick OTB	

123

12-Week General Prep/Base Phase

Week		MON	TUE	WED	THU	FRI	SAT	SUN
7	AM	Optional Swim: 30-60: Z2-3, Form	Key Bike I: 65: 10 Z4 (5), 4X2 Z5 (2)	Key Swim I: 40: Z4	Bike: 55: 30 SST	Key Swim E: 40-60 Z2-3	Key Bike E: 80: 3X10 Z4	Key Run E+I: 65: Z2 w/ 4X2 Z4 PUs
	PM	Optional Strength: 30	Run: 40: Z2	Run: 45: Z2 + strides	Strength: 30	Run: 45: Z2 + Strides	Run: 20 min Brick OTB	
8	AM	Optional Swim: 30-60 Z2-3, Form	Key Bike I: 65: 10 Z4 (5), 20 SST,	Key Swim I: 40: Z4	Bike: 50: 10X1 Z4, Alt Cadence	Key Swim E: 40-60: Z2-3	Key Bike E: 75: 4X10 Z3 (3)	Key Run E: 60: Z2 Hilly Course
	PM	Optional Strength: 30	Run: 40: Z2	Run: 40: Z2 + Strides	Strength: 30	Run: 45: Z2 + strides	Run: 20 min Brick OTB	
9	AM	Optional Swim: 30-60: Z2-3, Form	Key Bike I: 65: 7X3 Z5 (3)	Key Swim I: 40: Z4	Bike: 65: 45 mid to high Z3	Key Swim E: 40-60 Z2-3	Key Bike E: 75: 3X12 Z4 (3)	Key Run E+I: 70: Z2, 15 min Z4
	PM	Optional Strength: 30	Run: 40: Z2	Run: 45: Z2 + strides	Strength: 30	Run: 45: Z2 + Strides	Run: 20 min Brick OTB	
10	AM	Optional Swim: 30-60 Z2-3, Form	Key Bike I: 70: 2X20 SST (5)	Key Swim I: 40: Z4	Bike:70: 2X(5-4-3-2-1) Z4-5 (2-3)	Key Swim E: 40-60: Z2-3	Key Bike E: 85:6X5 Z4 (3)	Key Run E+I: 75: Z2 Hilly Course
	PM	Optional Strength: 30	Run: 40: Z2	Run: 50: Z2 + Strides	Strength: 30	Run: 45: Z2 + strides	Run: 20 min Brick OTB	
11	AM	Optional Swim: 30-60: Z2-3, Form	Key Bike I: 65: 3X10 Z4 (3)	Key Swim I: 40: Z4	Bike: 65: 3X10 SST, 2X5 Z4 (3)	Key Swim E: 40-60 Z2-3	Key Bike E: 90: 8X2 Z4-5, 8 min Z3 rec	Key Run E: 80: Z2, 20 min upper Z3
	PM	Optional Strength: 30	Run: 40: Z2	Run: 45: Z2 + strides	Strength: 30	Run: 45: Z2 + Strides	Run: 20 min Brick OTB	
12	AM	Optional Swim: 30-60 Z2-3, Form	Key Bike I: 50-70: 6X5 Z4 (2)	Key Swim I: 40: Z4	Bike: 50: Cad 6X(2 Z3 low, 2 Z4 high) (2)	Key Swim E: 40-60: Z2-3	Key Bike E: 85:30 min OU SST	Key Run E+I: 75: Z2, 4X1:30 Z4 PUs
	PM	Optional Strength: 30	Run: 40: Z2	Run: 45: Z2 + Strides	Strength: 30	Run: 45: Z2 + strides	Run: 20 min Brick OTB	

12-Week Half Iron Race Specific Plan

The following 12-week Half Iron Race Specific Plan covers the Specific Preparation Subphase and Competition Phase of training (i.e., the main build, peak and taper). You can acquire this and other TrainingPeaks formatted training plans by visiting. www.workingtriathlete.com.

A few highlights:

-Only begin this plan after developing a solid base of fitness.

-Like with the General Preparation Plan, this plan is structured so that you can adjust it to the time you have available to train, with optional workouts and opportunities to extend the duration. Always emphasize the main-set. If you are time-strapped, feel free to cut down the warm-up and cool-down. The exception to this rule is for the key endurance sessions, where overall volume/duration is important. Complete those workouts as prescribed.

-This plan is designed in four-week mesocycles, with three build weeks and one recovery week during which fatigue is unloaded. The plan culminates with a two-week taper leading to a Half Iron race.

12-Week Half Iron Specific

Week		MON	TUE	WED	THU	FRI	SAT	SUN
1	AM	Optional Swim: 30-60: Z2-3, Form	Key Bike I: 60: 3X10 Z4 (3)	Key Swim I: 40: Z3-Z4	Key Run I: 55: Cruise Intervals 4X5 Z4 (1)	Bike: 55: Middle 30 SST	Key Run E:90: 20 Z3-4 second half	Key Bike E: 2:00: 5X(5 SST, 1 Z4) (10)
	PM	Optional Strength: 30	Run: 30: Z2	Run: 40: Z2 + Strides	Strength: 30		Key Swim E: 40-60 Z2-3	Run: 20 min Brick OTB
2	AM	Optional Swim: 30-60 Z2-3, Form	Key Bike I: 50-70: 5X4 Z5 115% FTP (4)	Key Swim I: 40: Z3-Z4	Key Run I: 50: 8X1:30 Z5 (2)	Bike: 60:3X2 Cadence, 3X(5@85%, 5@95%) (3)	Key Run E:95: Z2 w/ 4X2 Z4-5 PUs	Key Bike E: 2:00 hrs: 4X2 Z4 (3), 60 Z3
	PM	Optional Strength: 30		Run: 40: Z2 + Strides	Strength: 30		Key Swim E: 40-60: Z2-3	Run: 20 min Brick OTB
3	AM	Optional Swim: 30-60: Z2-3, Form	Key Bike I: 55-70: 2X15 Z4 (5)	Key Swim I: 30: Z3-Z4	Key Run I: 50-60: 4X6 102% THR (~10K pace) (3)	Bike: 60-70: 5X(5 SST, 1 min high Z5) (4)	Key Run E:90: Z2 Run on a hilly route	Key Bike E: 2:00: 2X30 SST
	PM	Optional Strength: 30	Run: 30: Z2	Run: 40: Z2 + Strides	Strength: 30		Key Swim E: 40-60 Z2-3	Run: 20 min Brick OTB
4	AM	Optional Swim: 30-60 Z2-3, Form	Key Bike I: 65: 2X10 Z3, 2X10 SST (3)	Key Swim I: 30: Z3-Z4	Key Run I: 50: 20 min Z4 tempo	Bike: 45: 30 mid to upper Z3	Key Run E:80: Z2. 6X(20 sec Z5, 40 sec Z2)	Key Bike E: 1:45:30 min over under SST
	PM	Optional Strength: 30	Run: 30: Z2	Run: 40: Z2 + Strides	Strength: 30		Key Swim E: 40-60: Z2-3	Run: 20 min Brick OTB
5	AM	Optional Swim: 30-60: Z2-3, Form	Key Bike I: 70: 15 Z4 (5), 2X10 low Z5 (5)	Key Swim I: 40: Z3-Z4	Key Run I: 55: 5X3 5K pace (Z5) 3 min rec	Bike: 65: 25 SST (5), 10X1 110%/Z5 (1)	Key Run E: 1:40: Z2. 4X2 Z3-4 PUs	Key Bike E: 2:30-3:00: 6X5 SST (2)
	PM	Optional Strength: 30	Run: 30: Z2	Run: 30: Z2 + Strides	Strength: 30		Key Swim E: 40-60 Z2-3	Run: 20 min Brick OTB
6	AM	Optional Swim: 30-60 Z2-3, Form	Key Bike I: 65-85: 6X4 Z5 115% FTP (4)	Key Swim I: 40: Z3-Z4	Key Run I: 60: 30 min Z4 tempo	Bike: 60: 5X(3 Z3, 2 Z4) (2)	Key Run E: 1:50: Z2. Focus on good cadence.	Key Bike E: 2:30-3 hrs: Z2 3, 2X20 Z4 (5)
	PM	Optional Strength: 30	Run: 35: Z2	Run: 45: Z2 + Strides	Strength: 30		Key Swim E: 40-60: Z2-3	Run: 20 min Brick OTB

12-Week Half Iron Specific

Week		MON	TUE	WED	THU	FRI	SAT	SUN
7	AM	Optional Swim: 30-60: Z2-3, Form	Key Bike I: 75: 3X15 Z4 (3)	Key Swim I: 40: Z3-Z4	Key Run I: 65: 3X12 Z4 (2)	Bike: 60: 3X10 SST (2)	Key Run E: 1:40-2:00 hrs: Z2. Vary terrain.	Key Bike E: 2:30-3 hrs: 2X30 Z3
	PM	Optional Strength: 30	Run: 35: Z2	Run: 45: Z2 + Strides	Strength: 30		Key Swim E: 40-60 Z2-3	Run: 20 min Brick OTB
8	AM	Optional Swim: 30-60 Z2-3, Form	Key Bike I: 65: 1X10 SST, 1X15 Z4, 1X10 SST (1)	Key Swim I: 40: Z3-Z4	Key Run I:55: Cruise Intervals 5X5 Z4 (1)	Bike: 65: 5X(5 min high SST 90%, 1 min Z5 120%) (3)	Key Run E:70: Z2. Focus on good cadence.	Key Bike E: 1:45:30 min over under SST (5 min 94%, 5 min 85% FTP)
	PM	Optional Strength: 30	Run: 30: Z2	Run: 35: Z2 + Strides	Strength: 30		Key Swim E: 40-60: Z2-3	Run: 20 min Brick OTB
9	AM	Optional Swim: 30-60: Z2-3, Form	Key Bike I: 70: 8X3 min Z5 (2)	Key Swim I: 40: Z3-Z4	Key Run I: 60: 6-5-4-3-2-1 min, Z5 ascending (2-3)	Bike: 60: 1X20 Z3 (80%), 1X15 SST (85%)	Key Run E:1:40: Z2, last 20 min build to tempo	Key Bike E: 2:40: (Z3 80-82%) for 2:00-2:30
	PM	Optional Strength: 30	Run: 35: Z2	Run: 40: Z2 + Strides	Strength: 30		Key Swim E: 40-60 Z2-3	Run: 30 min Brick OTB
10	AM	Optional Swim: 30-60 Z2-3, Form	Key Bike I: 55: 5X(4 SST, 1 Z5) (2)	Key Swim I: 40: Z3-Z4	Key Run I: 35: 25 min Z3-Z4 Tempo	Bike: 60: 40 OU SST	Key Run E:80: Z2 with 4X1:30 Z5 in middle	Key Bike E: 2:20: 3X15 SST (5)
	PM	Optional Strength: 30	Run: 35: Z2	Run: 40: Z2 + Strides	Strength: 30		Key Swim E: 40-60: Z2-3	Run: 20 min Brick OTB
11	AM	Optional Swim: 30-60: Z2-3, Form	Key Bike I: 65: 1X15 SST, 2X4 Z5 (4)	Key Swim I: 40: Z3-Z4	Key Run I: 55: 4X3 min Z4-5 PU	Bike: 60: 2X15 100% FTP (5)	Key Run E:70: Z2. 4X2 min Z3-4 PUs	Key Bike E: 1:40: 4X(5 min SST, 1 Z5 110 RPM)(3)
	PM		Run: 35: Z2	Run: 40: Z2 + Strides			Key Swim E: 40-60 Z2-3	Run: 20 min Brick OTB
12	AM	Optional Swim: 30-60 Z2-3, Form	Bike: 45: 4X1:30 Z4 (3)	Key Swim I: 40: Z3-Z4	Run: 30: Z2, 4x1 Z3-4 (2)	Swim: 10 min 4X30 sec builds Bike: 15 min bike check, 2X30 sec builds	RACE	
	PM		Run: 35: Z2, 4x1 min Z4 PUs	Bike: 40: 3X1:30 Z4(3)		Run: 15: 3X1 min builds		

Works Cited

Boutcher, Stephen H. "High-Intensity Intermittent Exercise and Fat Loss." Journal of Obesity, Hindawi Publishing Corporation, 24 Nov. 2010, www.ncbi.nlm.nih.gov/pmc/articles/PMC2991639/.

Burgomaster, K A, et al. "Similar Metabolic Adaptations during Exercise after Low Volume Sprint Interval and Traditional Endurance Training in Humans." The Journal of Physiology., U.S. National Library of Medicine, 1 Jan. 2008, www.ncbi.nlm.nih.gov/pubmed/17991697.

CostillDL, FlynnMG, Kirman JP, et al. Effects of repeated daysof intensified training on muscle glycogen and swimming performance. Med Sci Sports Exerc 1988; 20: 249-54.

Damasceno, M V, et al. "Effects of Resistance Training on Neuromuscular Characteristics and Pacing during 10-Km Running Time Trial." European Journal of Applied Physiology., U.S. National Library of Medicine, July 2015, www.ncbi.nlm.nih.gov/pubmed/25697149.

Daussin, F N, et al. "Effect of Interval versus Continuous Training on Cardiorespiratory and Mitochondrial Functions: Relationship to Aerobic Performance Improvements in Sedentary Subjects." American Journal of Physiology. Regulatory, Integrative and Comparative Physiology., U.S. National Library of Medicine, July 2008, www.ncbi.nlm.nih.gov/pubmed/18417645.

Fleck, S J, and J E Falkel. "Value of Resistance Training for the Reduction of Sports Injuries." Sports Medicine (Auckland, N.Z.)., U.S. National Library of Medicine, Jan. 1986, www.ncbi.nlm.nih.gov/pubmed/3633121.

Helgerud, J, et al. "Aerobic High-Intensity Intervals Improve VO2max More than Moderate Training." Medicine and Science in Sports and Exercise., U.S. National Library of Medicine, Apr. 2007, www.ncbi.nlm.nih.gov/pubmed/17414804.

Londeree BR. Effect of training on lactate/ventilatory thresholds: a meta-analysis. Med Sci Sports Exerc 1997; 29: 837-43.

McGehee, J C, et al. "A Comparison of Methods for Estimating the Lactate Threshold."Journal of Strength and Conditioning Research., U.S. National Library of Medicine, Aug. 2005, www.ncbi.nlm.nih.gov/pubmed/16095403.

Støren, O, et al. "Maximal Strength Training Improves Running Economy in Distance Runners." Medicine and Science in Sports and Exercise., U.S. National Library of Medicine, June 2008, www.ncbi.nlm.nih.gov/pubmed/18460997.

Trapp EG, Chisholm DJ, Freund J, Boutcher SH. The effects of high-intensity intermittent exercise training on fat loss and fasting insulin levels of young women. International Journal of Obesity. 2008;32(4):684–691.

Weston AR, Myburgh KH, Lindsay FH, et al. Skeletal muscle buffering capacity and endurance performance after high intensity training by well-trained cyclists. European Journal of Applied Physiology and Occupational Physiology 1997; 75: 7-13

About the author:

Conrad Goeringer is an Ironman Certified Coach based out of Nashville, TN. He is a multi-time triathlon champion and USAT National Duathlon Champion. His passion is helping athletes of all levels and with all schedules achieve their endurance goals. To learn more about joining the Working Triathlete community, visit www.workingtriathlete.com *and reach out for a free consultation.*

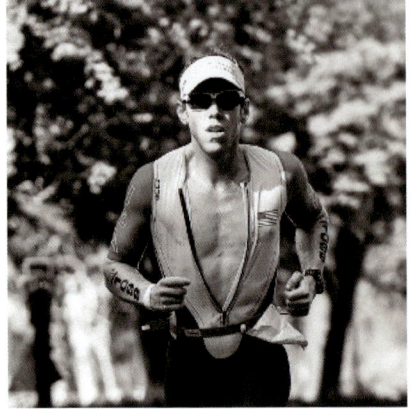

WT WORKING TRIATHLETE

www.workingtriathlete.com

45137779R00077

Printed in Poland
by Amazon Fulfillment
Poland Sp. z o.o., Wrocław